Christiana Maria Ribeiro Salles Vanni

Pectoralis Major Myocutaneous Flap in Head and Neck Surgery

Christiana Maria Ribeiro Salles Vanni

Pectoralis Major Myocutaneous Flap in Head and Neck Surgery

Anatomical Study in Reconstruction

ScienciaScripts

Imprint
Any brand names and product names mentioned in this book are subject to trademark, brand or patent protection and are trademarks or registered trademarks of their respective holders. The use of brand names, product names, common names, trade names, product descriptions etc. even without a particular marking in this work is in no way to be construed to mean that such names may be regarded as unrestricted in respect of trademark and brand protection legislation and could thus be used by anyone.

Cover image: www.ingimage.com

This book is a translation from the original published under ISBN 978-3-330-76512-2.

Publisher:
Sciencia Scripts
is a trademark of
Dodo Books Indian Ocean Ltd. and OmniScriptum S.R.L publishing group

120 High Road, East Finchley, London, N2 9ED, United Kingdom
Str. Armeneasca 28/1, office 1, Chisinau MD-2012, Republic of Moldova, Europe
Managing Directors: Ieva Konstantinova, Victoria Ursu
info@omniscriptum.com

Printed at: see last page
ISBN: 978-620-8-51598-0

SUMMARY

SUMMARY

Vanni CMRS. *MAJOR PECTAL MIOCUTANEOUS RETAIL IN THE RECONSTRUCTION OF HEAD AND NECK DEFECTS: AN ANATOMICAL STUDY* [thesis]. São Paulo: Department of Surgery, Faculty of Medicine, University of São Paulo; 2013.

Objectives: To assess whether the length of the pedicle of the pectoralis major myocutaneous flap and its reach to various sites in the cervicofacial region are influenced by anthropometric data and the side on which the flap is dissected. The study also aims to determine whether infraclavicular rotation provides a significant gain in flap reach compared to supraclavicular rotation.
Design: Prospective anatomical cross-sectional study of cadavers and patients.
Materials: 50 pectoralis major myocutaneous flaps were studied in 25 non-formalised adult cadavers less than 24 hours after death, provided by the University of São Paulo's Death Verification Service, and then 15 patients who underwent reconstruction of cervicofacial defects with this flap.
Methods: In all the cases studied, a quadrangular skin island measuring 8x6 cm (height x width) was standardised, located over the sternocostal portion of the pectoralis major muscle, medially to the nipple and with the upper edge of the seventh rib as its caudal limit. All the flaps were based only on the pectoral branch of the thoracoacromial artery and the rotation was carried out initially over the clavicle. The length of the pedicle was measured after rotation, from the clavicular midpoint to the level of the upper edge of the skin island. The reach of the centre of the flap's skin island was tested for the following regions: laryngeal prominence of the thyroid cartilage, chin, angle of the mandible, external auditory canal and orbit. The relationship between the length of the pedicle and the reach of the flap with anthropometric data and the side of dissection was analysed. Subsequently, the flap was rotated under the clavicle only in the cadavers and its reach was tested again for the same regions, comparing it with the results of supraclavicular rotation.
Results: In the cadavers, the length of the pedicle showed an average value of 17.67 ± 2.24 cm, while for the patients, we found an average of 16.03 ± 1.35 cm. All the flaps reached all the regions studied, with the exception of the orbit, which was reached in cadavers in 20 cases by supraclavicular rotation (40%) and 21 cases by infraclavicular rotation (42%). In patients, the orbit was reached in 13.3% of cases. In cadavers, infraclavicular rotation showed no significant gain in reaching the orbit (p=0.839 - chi-squared) or in the other regions studied, although there was a gain of 0.61 cm in the average length of the pedicle, which was statistically significant (p=0.01; by Person's Correlation). Considering the cadavers, the univariate analysis showed that there was a statistically significant difference in the flap's reach to the orbit in individuals with a greater acromion-trochanteric distance - ATD (p= 0.008 - Student's t-test), greater biacromial distance - DBA (p= 0.024 - Student's t-test) and lower ratio of mastoid to sternal furcula distance - DMF/DAT (p= 0.005 - Student's t-test). It was also observed that cadavers whose flaps reached the orbit were statistically heavier (p=0.036 - Student's t-test). With regard to the length of the pedicle, in the univariate analysis, there was a positive and statistically significant correlation between the length of the pedicle and the biacromial distance (r= 0.311; p= 0.028 - Pearson's correlation); negative correlation and also significant with the ratio between the mastoid-sternal furcula distance and the biacromial distance - DMF/DBA (r= - 0.362; p= 0.010 - Pearson's correlation) and with the ratio between the mastoid-sternal furcula distance and the acromion-trochanteric distance - DMF/DAT (r= - 0.403; p= 0.004 - Pearson's correlation). As for the patients, the univariate analysis showed a positive and statistically significant correlation between the

length of the pedicle and the length of the sternum - CE (r= 0.722; p= 0.002 - Sperman's correlation) and a negative and also significant correlation with the ratio between the mastoid-sternal furcula distance and the length of the sternum - DMF/CE (r= -0.587; p= 0.021 - Sperman's correlation). With the results obtained in this last analysis, the variables in the patients with $p<0.20$ were subjected to multivariate analysis using a linear regression model, with the aim of establishing the variables that can determine the length of the flap's vascular pedicle. In this way, the length of the sternum was identified as the only variable capable of determining the length of the vascular pedicle of the PMVR (p=0.004). Based on this regression data, an equation was established to determine the length of the vascular pedicle of the PMVR (COMP) based on the length of the sternum, as shown below: COMP = 2.54 + 0.64 X CE.

Conclusions: Infraclavicular rotation of the pectoralis major myocutaneous flap does not provide a gain in flap reach to the cervicofacial region compared to supraclavicular rotation; the reach of the pectoralis major myocutaneous flap is not influenced by the side of dissection and anthropometric data; the length of the vascular pedicle is not influenced by the side of dissection, but is positively influenced by sternal length. Although the length of the flap is not influenced by anthropometric data, this anatomical model suggests that the equation determining the length of the pedicle can, in clinical practice, contribute to the planning of reconstructions using the pectoralis major myocutaneous flap, especially for more cranial defects.

Keywords: 1- Surgical flaps 2- Reconstructive surgical procedures 3- Head and neck neoplasms 4- Anatomy 5- Cadaver.

CHAPTER 1

INTRODUCTION

The reconstruction of complex defects in head and neck surgery is still a challenge for surgeons. At the end of the 1970s, following the anatomical description of myocutaneous perforating vessels, the use of myocutaneous or musculocutaneous flaps became more popular, having been used sporadically in the past, especially since the beginning of the 20th century(1, 2). Another factor that made the use of these flaps more common was the evidence of an axial vascularisation pattern found in some muscles, which allows them to be transposed by means of an arc of rotation or microsurgical anastomosis of their vascular pedicle(3). These anatomical characteristics make these flaps reliable and versatile for complex reconstructions(4).

Perhaps the area of head and neck surgery that has seen the greatest advances in the last 50 years is reconstruction, due to the description of a series of pedicled and free flaps(5-10). Nowadays, it can be said that there is no defect that cannot be repaired, and this gives the surgeon a greater margin of safety to carry out a safe and truly oncological resection. The head and neck region has peculiarities in its intrinsic form and function, and careful reconstruction is necessary to return the patient to their pre-morbid condition. The functions of phonation, swallowing and aesthetics are most commonly focussed on when considering rehabilitation objectives. Once the oncological resection has been carried out and its consequent surgical defect established, the surgeon is faced with the challenge of maintaining a balance between the airway, phonation, swallowing and aesthetics, occasionally having to weigh up and compromise(11) one function in order to improve another(12).

Aesthetic deformities are most evident in the head and neck region. Generally speaking, the principles include reconstructing the underlying bone structure, replacing dry skin with skin of a corresponding quality and appearance, minimising the visibility of scars and retractions, and reconstructing in areas of the facial units. The skin should be of corresponding colour, thickness and hair-bearing units, where possible. Facial units include the forehead, eyes and periorbital area, mid-face, nose (and its subunits), lips and chin. There are a range of reconstruction options, such as healing by second intention and primary closure on one spectrum, and complex reconstructions with free flaps on the opposite spectrum.

The reconstructive option selected depends on the following factors: the location and extent of the defect; the patient's general health; existing and available donor areas for making flaps; the condition of the tissue adjacent to the defect (irradiated, infected, previously operated on); and the functionality of the area to be reconstructed. Not only must the surgeon choose which option is best for a given defect, but secondary and tertiary options must be studied and planned in the event of flap failure or recurrent disease.

Closure by second intention is an excellent option in various clinical scenarios, such as mucosal defects with a preserved muscular underlying layer. In general, primary closure is the most commonly used option for closing small defects. Attempts should be made to keep the incisions within relaxed skin tension lines; these lines are caused by muscle insertion into the skin and form when mimetic movement occurs. Incisions parallel to the relaxed skin tension lines not only respect the aesthetic units of the face, but also have the least amount of tension along them, which reduces scarring. The zetaplasty technique can be used to reorient an unfavourable closure line to a relaxed skin tension line. This technique, described more than 150 years ago, is used because of its ability to lengthen linear scars, using relatively loose adjacent tissue(13).

Skin grafts are most commonly used in the oral cavity, ear or maxillectomy defects, as well as to cover flap donor areas such as the antebrachial free flap, deltopectoral flap and temporofrontal flap. Skin grafts are completely dependent on the nutrition of the tissue on which they are placed and can evolve well on muscle, perichondrium and periosteum. They should not be used on bone or cartilage without periosteum or perichondrium, nor on tissues that have been irradiated or are infected.

Local skin flaps have excellent tissue correspondence due to their proximity to the defect. They are commonly used in the reconstruction of lip and facial skin defects, and the most commonly used are the nasolabial, rhomboid and bilobed, median frontal and Mustardé flaps(14-17). Similar to primary closure, local flaps must have a design to be incorporated into the skin's tension lines. Many of these local flaps have random vascularisation, dependent on the subdermal capillary plexus, which makes their width/length ratio important for maintaining viability. Others, such as the median frontal flap, popularly known as the Indian flap, are axial, i.e. they have a well-defined vascular pedicle contained in the subcutaneous fascia or in an underlying muscle.

The post-excisional defect of an oral tumour, for example, depending on its location and size, can be closed primarily with a simple suture. However, when resecting larger lesions, primary reconstruction is often not possible, either because it is impossible to directly approach the free edges of the defect, or because the mobility of the structures to be sutured is compromised. Therefore, in order to adequately repair the defect and preserve the function of the organs to be reconstructed, it is necessary to mobilise neighbouring or distant tissues to the region of the defect. In this context, the surgeon has free flaps and some local and regional pedicled flap options available(18).

1.1. HISTORY OF HEAD AND NECK RECONSTRUCTIVE SURGERY

Head and neck reconstructive surgery has come a long way since the speciality was first established. In the 1940s, cervical skin flaps were used at various surgical stages to rehabilitate treated patients. A classic example of these flaps is the Wookey flap, used to reconstruct the pharyngo-oesophageal transit after pharyngolaryngectomies.(19) From the

1960s onwards, a series of pedicled flaps were described, giving great impetus to reconstructive surgery in the head and neck. This was followed by microsurgical flaps developed from the 1980s onwards, which are currently considered the gold standard in cervicofacial reconstruction. The following paragraphs discuss the main flaps used in the speciality, with special attention to the pectoralis major myocutaneous flap.

1.1.1. MEDIAN FRONTAL FLAP

The first mention of head and neck reconstruction refers to the median frontal flap, also known as the Indian flap. Sushruta Samhita was an important 6th century BC physician from the city of Varanas, India. The texts that have been preserved date back to the 3rd and 4th centuries AD. Considered one of the fathers of traditional Indian Ayurvedic medicine, he presents in Charaka Samhita, which would have been the compendium of medicine at the time, descriptions of diseases, medicines, treatments, surgical techniques and human anatomy. Sushruta Samhita is considered the father of plastic surgery for his initial descriptions of defects and how to repair them. His great achievement in this area was post-amputation nasal reconstruction as a punishment for adulterers(20-22). This flap is pedicled to the supratrochlear and possibly supraorbital vessels, and usually requires two surgical times to complete the proposed reconstruction.

Specifically in nasal reconstruction, other names stood out, such as Gustavo Branca and Tagliacozzi, who used local flaps and the medial arm flap, respectively. However, it was Johann F. Dieffenbach, born in Germany in 1792, who developed most of the flaps for reconstructive rhinoplasty. Among the techniques developed by his successors are the classic frontal flap, oblique frontal flap, supratrochlear or paramedian flap, Converse flap, Washio flap, Orticochea flap, nasogenian subcutaneous pedicle flap and the Rintalla flap(23-26).

1.1.2. LATISSIMUS DORSI MYOCUTANEOUS FLAP

In 1896, Tansini described the pedicled flap of the latissimus dorsi muscle, the first myocutaneous flap reported in medical literature. This flap was used to reconstruct the chest wall after extended radical mastectomy. In 1978, Quillen made the first description of the use of this pedicled flap in the head and neck, for reconstruction of the jugal mucosa after resection of a recurrent tumour. After that, the technique became popularised for the use of the latissimus dorsi as a pedicled or free flap (27-31).

1.1.3. SUPRACLAVICULAR FLAP

In 1949, Kazanjian and Converse made the first description of the fasciocutaneous shoulder flap or acromial flap with random vascularisation, since initially there was no knowledge of the vascular supply(32). A few years later, its use was chosen almost exclusively for the treatment of cervical contractures. Its advantages are that it is thin and has the same colour as the area of skin to be reconstructed, its arc of rotation is located in the neck, which provides great reach, and the donor area can be closed primarily, which reduces surgical time(33). The supraclavicular pedicle originates from the transverse cervical vessels and was described and studied for the first time in 1978, along with the anatomy of the shoulder. Initially accepted as a cervicoumeral flap, the vascular pedicle is located in the triangle limited by the posterior margin of the sternocleidomastoid muscle, the external jugular vein and the upper edge of the clavicle. The flap can measure 10 to 16 cm in width and 22 to 30 cm in length(34, 35). Around the 1980s, after the description of the trapezial flap and the advent of the pectoralis major myocutaneous flap, associated with some shortcomings of the supraclavicular flap, such as necrosis of the distal portion, dehiscence of the donor area, this flap was forgotten. However, since 2000, some authors have re-established its interest and use in head and neck oncological reconstructions, and it can currently be considered one of the most widely used in certain services(36). Alves et al. refer to the supraclavicular flap as a new reconstructive option after resections of extensive cutaneous tumours in the head and neck(37).

1.1.4. TEMPOROFRONTAL FLAP

Described by McGregor in 1963 for the reconstruction of intraoral defects, the temporofrontal flap or frontal flap with temporal base is a pedicled myocutaneous flap irrigated by the superficial temporal artery, a branch of the external carotid artery. The flap is composed of the skin of the frontal region and the underlying frontal muscle, and its viability is maintained by a temporary or definitive vascular connection. After its initial description, this flap began to be used for a large number of reconstructions in the head and neck segment, such as the orbital cavity, genital region, jugal mucosa and floor of the mouth. The major disadvantage related to its use is the aesthetic deformity in the patient's donor area, which necessarily needs to be grafted. Although considered by many to be of historical value only in exceptional situations where other reconstruction options are not possible, the McGregor frontal flap is still a safe and effective alternative for repairing complex defects involving the face and oral cavity(38-43).

1.1.5. DELTOPECTORAL FLAP

Also in the 1960s, the deltopectoral cutaneous fascia flap, also referred to as the Bakamjian flap, based on the perforating arteries of the first four intercostal branches of the internal thoracic artery, was the greatest advance in head and neck surgery at the time. It was initially used as an alternative for reconstructing circular hypopharyngeal defects after pharyngolaryngectomy(44). There is some controversy over the initial description of this flap. It is speculated that it was first mentioned in 1917 by Aymard for nasal reconstruction. It was described for the second time in the 1930s by Joseph in his book on plastic surgery, and referred to Manchot's description of the vascular territory and supply of this flap(45, 46). For approximately forty years, this flap remained forgotten in the medical literature until Bakamjian described it in Head and Neck Reconstruction, talking about the flap's versatility and wide application(28, 47). This flap was one of the first regional flaps and has been used extensively in head and neck reconstruction. From an anatomical point of view, it has a medial base and is drawn over the upper regions of the pectoral and deltoid muscles. Due to the flexibility of the transferred skin, it can be used either for neck skin defects or folded back on itself for pharyngeal reconstruction. A very wide skin flap that has undergone previous autonomisation can be transferred to reconstruct defects up to the rhinopharynx. The donor area can be made up of a large portion of skin from the deltoid region that has not undergone radiotherapy in previous treatments, or with previous incisions from the resection of the initial lesion, or even the final portion of the pedicle of the pectoralis major myocutaneous flap.

1.1.6. TRAPEZIUS MYOCUTANEOUS FLAPS

The design of this flap was first developed by Mútter (48) in 1842 and later by Zovickian (49) in 1957. These two authors used the skin flap respectively to correct burn scars and later to correct pharyngeal fistulas. A myocutaneous flap was created in 1972 by Conley(50), who included the muscles of the upper trapezius and the clavicular portion, a technique that became known as the upper trapezial myocutaneous flap. Seven years later, Demergasso and Piazza described the trapezial myocutaneous flap made up of the trapezial muscle based on the transverse cervical artery, as the name suggests(51) and became known as the lateral trapezial myocutaneous flap. The myocutaneous flap of the lower part of the trapezius, known as the inferior or posterior trapezial flap, was described in 1980 by Baek et al.(52) based on the dorsal scapular artery and also the territory of the transverse cervical artery, and has already been mentioned as an excellent choice for lateral temporal bone defects(50, 53, 54). In addition to reconstructing mucosal defects with vascularised skin, covering the exposed carotid artery is an excellent indication for this flap. The posterior vertical trapezius myocutaneous flap is the technique of choice in selected cases for closing defects in the occipital, parotid (lateral facial), posterior cervical and upper third of the thoracic dorsum regions. Its use is somewhat restricted because it requires a change of decubitus, and there are other options with similar results(55-57).

The flap is made up of a large, triangular, bilateral and symmetrical muscle, located on the thoracic dorsum, which can be divided anatomically into three thirds: upper, middle and lower and is innervated by the XI cranial nerve, the accessory spinal nerve. Classically, myocutaneous flaps are classified according to the type of vascularisation. In this case, it is classified by Mathew-Nahai as type II, i.e. with vascularisation by a dominant pedicle, which is the descending branch of the transverse cervical artery, and several smaller secondary pedicles, posterior intercostal perforators. Later, other authors(8, 58, 59) demonstrated a new vascular pattern, with the dominant nourishing vessel being the dorsal scapular artery, thus having two dominant pedicles . The functions of this muscle are: maintaining the shoulder in an anatomical position, helping with its elevation and rotation (mainly the upper third) and bringing the scapulae closer to the midline (the middle third). As seen above, the trapezius muscle offers multiple soft tissue flaps that can be rotated for defects in the head and neck.

1.1.7. TEMPOROPARIETAL GALEAL FLAP

Among the options and diversity of flaps described and used for the cervicofacial region, the temporoparietal galeal flap is described, as its name implies, as a flap made from the galeal tissue of the temporoparietal region. The temporoparietal fascia and aponeurotic galea is a thin, malleable tissue, extremely vascularised by the superficial temporal, supratrochlear, supraorbital and occipital vessels, and is made up of dense connective tissue. It rests just below the hair follicles and subcutaneous tissue, to which it adheres loosely just above the zygomatic arch. This flap was first described by Fox and Edgerton(60) for ear reconstruction, but its use was extended to other regions, including intraoral defects.

Its rotation under the zygomatic arch can provide reach to the base of the tongue, contralateral floor and cervical carotid coverage. Around the beginning of the 21st century, the temporoparietal galeal flap pedicled on the superficial temporal vessels was described for facial reconstruction in the oral cavity and oropharynx after successful resection of malignant tumours(61). Its rotation below the zygomatic arches can provide reach to the base of the tongue, contra lateral floor and cervical carotid coverage(62-64). Despite the few reports in the literature, the results of its use in intraoral defects seem to be satisfactory, with low complication rates including transient alopecia of the donor area in some patients.

1.1.8. FREE FLAPS

Free or microsurgical flaps, considered the "gold standard" for head and neck reconstruction, are not available in many centres that treat cancer in this location due to the high costs and highly specialised technology associated with these flaps(65). In addition, the generally longer anaesthetic time associated with microsurgical flaps(18) makes this type of reconstruction unsuitable for patients with low *performance status* or many clinical comorbidities. With the increase in the number of patients with head and neck cancer who are initially treated with chemotherapy and high doses of radiotherapy, there has been an increase in the number of salvage surgeries. In these surgeries, it is common to see poor quality recipient cervical vessels due to previous treatments, particularly radiotherapy, which also makes the use of microsurgical flaps unfeasible in many cases. For these reasons, pedicled flaps remain important in many oncology institutions in Brazil and around the world, and are still used on a large scale in various centres and the subject of many publications(47, 55, 62, 66-71).

However, tumours that used to be considered unresectable, due to the extensive involvement of soft tissues and deep bone structures, can now be safely removed with wide and safe resection margins, thanks to new and efficient reconstruction techniques. The result of these wide-ranging tumour ablations are complex, large, three-dimensional defects associated with bone exposure, meningeal exposure and brain parenchyma. Therefore, microsurgical transplantation is a very important part of the treatment, as it provides richly vascularised tissue to fill, support and isolate the bone structures, allowing the meninges and brain tissue to be separated from the oral and nasal cavities, thus preventing high morbidity complications such as skull base osteomyelitis, meningitis, brain abscess and, in parallel, less impairment of speech and swallowing with the patient's early return to social life when the surgery progresses well(72).

Among the most widely used free flaps in head and neck surgery, we can mention the antebrachial flap described in 1981 by Yang et al. in China, which is why it is also known as the "Chinese flap"(73), and which began to be widely used in the reconstruction of cervicofacial and craniofacial defects by Soutar and Mcgregor(74). There is also the anterolateral thigh flap, described by Song et al. in 1984 in the English literature(75) and, in parallel, by Luo et al. in 1985 in the Chinese literature(76, 77). This flap is nourished by perforating vessels from the descending or transverse branch of the lateral circumflex femoral artery. Another example is the rectus abdominis myocutaneous flap, which was first described in the literature in 1977 by Drever in the form of a vertical island(78, 79). In 1979, Robbins was the first to use the rectus flap for breast reconstruction(78, 80, 81). There is also the lateral arm flap(82, 83), fibula free flap(84) and jejunum free flap(85).

Each of these flaps has specific indications and many of them can be used to reconstruct the same type of defect, such as the free jejunum flap and the anterolateral thigh flap, which can be used to reconstruct circular pharyngeal defects(86-88). The choice of a particular flap is determined by the individual characteristics of the clinical case and the surgeon's experience(89).

1.2. PECTORALIS MAJOR MYOCUTANEOUS FLAP

Described by Stephan Ariyan in 1979(90) for its applicability in head and neck reconstructions, the pectoralis major myocutaneous flap (PMMF) is one of the most widely used in repairing defects in this region. As well as having the reliability of an axial musculocutaneous flap, its arc of rotation is suitable for reaching most cervicofacial defects and allows reconstruction in a single time with primary closure of the donor area(4, 91-93). The pectoralis major myocutaneous flap stands out not only in head and neck reconstructions, but also in the chest, back, upper limbs and also remotely (microsurgical). When using this muscle, a thorough knowledge of its anatomy and neighbouring regions is extremely important in order to familiarise oneself with these structures and ensure greater safety when handling it. Knowledge of the size and limits of the muscle, its vascular network and its relationship with neighbouring structures is of fundamental importance in order to be safe when making a flap.

1.2.1. HISTORY OF THE PECTORALIS MAJOR MUSCLE FLAP

The first report found in the literature using the pectoralis major muscle in reconstructions was described by Pickrell et al. (1947) in the repair of a chest wall defect after radical mastectomy(94). Thirty years later, Mcgraw et al. (1977) carried out anatomical studies of the pectoralis major muscle, defined territories of myocutaneous vascularisation and thus made it possible to use it as a myocutaneous island flap(95, 96). Brown et al.(97) added the possibility of using this muscle for the reconstruction of defects not only in the chest, but also in the lower neck. In 1977(98), Sisson et al. demonstrated not only the importance of using the pectoralis major muscle in laryngeal carcinoma peritracheostomy recurrence operations, but also, in addition to the mediastinal dissection and tracheal resection technique, the importance of filling the space created between the trachea and the aortic arch or between the trachea and the innominate artery with pectoralis major muscle flaps, transposed by advancement to the defect region.

Ariyan (1979) performed the first head and neck reconstruction using the pectoralis major muscle, standardising its use as a myocutaneous flap and describing its anatomy and surgical technique. The pectoralis major muscle has been used surgically in two ways(99): as a pedicled flap and a free flap(100). The pedicle-based muscle has been mobilised to repair deformities of the chest wall(101, 102), upper arm and elbow. The use of the free or microsurgical flap for distant reconstructions has been described in Japan and Canada.

Chaffai et al. (1988) carried out an anatomical study of the pectoralis major muscle with the aim of observing not only the vasculonervous supply of the clavicular and sternal costal portions in order to utilise them separately, but also the branches of the thoracoacromial artery that irrigate these structures separately, making it possible to utilise them in isolation(103). Bloch (1984) carried out a study on 40 anatomical specimens of the pectoralis major muscle and published the results, in which 75% showed a dominant pedicle of the thoracoacromial artery and in the other 25% there was dominance of two pedicles, one from the thoracoacromial artery and the other from the lateral thoracic artery(104). Viterbo et al. (1985) published a study on the anatomy of the pectoralis major muscle with vascular measurements, a study of the cutaneous territory and the arc of rotation(105).

1.2.2. SURGICAL ANATOMY

The thick pectoralis major muscle, also called the pectoralis major, covers the upper portion of each side of the chest in a fan shape due to its wide, triangular shape. On each side, it occupies the anterolateral wall of the chest wall, immediately deeper than the mammary gland, and reaches the concave portion of the armpit. Its main actions on the arm are medial rotation, powerful adduction, elevation and abduction, together with the shoulder. As a secondary function, this muscle elevates the upper ribs, throws and pushes the arm.

It has three fascicles that originate on the upper edge of the clavicle (clavicular fascicle), on the anterior face of the sternum and first costal arches (sternocostal fascicle) and on the lower costal arches and aponeurosis of the rectus abdominis muscle (abdominal fascicle or lateral). The clavicular fibres are normally separated from the sternal fibres by a small space through which the thoracoacromial artery can be identified as soon as it pierces the clavipeitoral fascia, on the anterior surface of the sternum and first costal arches (sternocostal fascicle) and in the lower costal arches and aponeurosis of the rectus abdominis muscle (abdominal or lateral fascicle). Its fibres converge and insert into the Christian of the greater tubercle of the humerus, where it inserts into the anterior lip of the bicipital groove forming a wide quadrilateral tendon. Therefore, the body of this muscle has three portions: clavicular, upper costal sternum and lower costal sternum, and in practice the only portion that differs from the others is the clavicular. Testut et al.(106) report that in around 35% of cases there is a possibility that the lower costal sternum portion is missing, and it can also be seen separately from the rest of the muscle or sometimes divided into two or three fascicles. The insertion into the bicipital groove can be made up of several well-defined supernumerary fascicles. The partial or total absence of this muscle can occur when it is usually accompanied by thoracic deformities(107), which is what happens in Poland's Syndrome, a rare congenital anomaly that has a risk of recurrence of less than 1% in the same family(108).

1.2.3. VASCULARISATION

Initially, Ariyan carried out an anatomical study on fresh cadavers in which he determined that the main vascular supply to the MPMR was derived from the thoracoacromial artery (or acromiothoracic artery) and that additional vascularisation to the muscle was derived from the superior thoracic and lateral thoracic arteries. The vascularisation of this muscle comes mainly from the pectoral branch of the thoracoacromial or acromiothoracic artery. This artery, despite being popularly described as a branch of the subclavian artery in Ariyan's work(109, 110), actually originates in the second portion of the axillary artery and therefore a little below the lower edge of the clavicle(111) as shown in Figure 1.

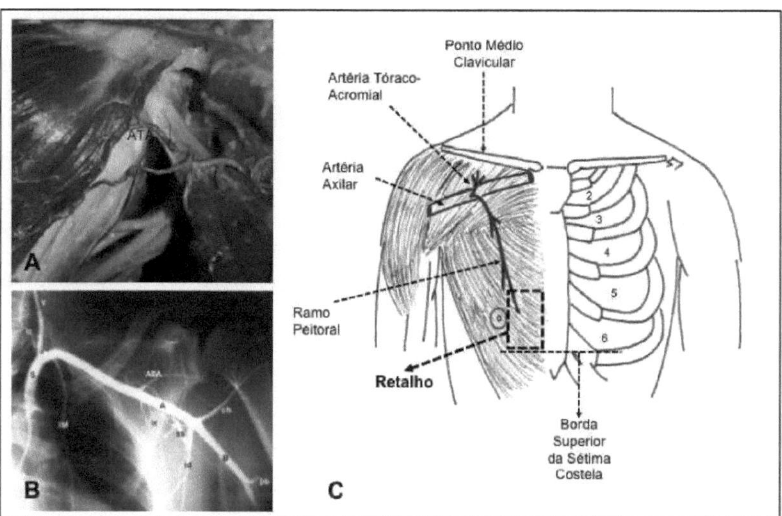

Figure 1. Anatomical dissection (A) and arteriography (B) of the scapular girdle, showing the emergence of the thoracoacromial artery (TAA) - reproduced with permission. Anatomical representation of the vascular pedicle and positioning of the pectoralis major myocutaneous flap (C).

The pectoral branch of the thoracoacromial artery, as shown, originates from the axillary artery and is considered the main arterial pedicle of the MPMR, primarily perfusing the sternocostal fascicle of the pectoralis major muscle. The secondary pedicles are the lateral thoracic, superior thoracic and internal thoracic arteries. The lateral thoracic artery of the muscle, a direct branch of the

The axillary artery is responsible for vascularising the lateral fascicle, while the clavicular fascicle is vascularised by the superior thoracic artery, which originates from the axillary artery. The internal artery is a branch of the subclavian artery, which has a descending parasternal and extrapleural course within the anterior chest wall and gives rise to the intercostal branches that follow the lower edge of the ribs. The intercostal branches of the

1st, 2nd and 3rd intercostal spaces give rise to perforating branches in a parasternal position that irrigate the skin of this region of the thorax, as well as the upper portion of the pectoralis major muscle, above the level of the 4th rib. These muscle perforating branches have a true anastomosis with the pectoral branch of the thoracoacromial artery, particularly the one originating from the 3rd intercostal perforating branch, giving rise to a rich vascular territory. At the level of the 4th, 5th ° and 6th intercostal spaces there is another vascular territory made up of several perforating branches of the internal thoracic artery and its intercostal branches that anastomose with each other(3, 112-118). According to Mathes and Nahai's vascular classification(119), this flap has a type V classification, i.e. it has a dominant pedicle and secondary vascular pedicles. The venous drainage of the pectoralis major muscle is via comitant veins that accompany the respective arteries.

1.2.4. INNOVATION

The motor innervation of this muscle consists of the lateral (greater) and medial (lesser) pectoral nerves, which originate respectively from C5 to C7 and from C8 to T1; in the brachial plexus, the clavicular segment receives branches exclusively from the lateral pectoral nerve, the sternocostal segment from both nerves and the abdominal or lower costal sternal segment from the medial pectoral nerve(120, 121). Resection of the pectoral nerve branches ensures muscle atrophy and reduces the volume over the clavicle after rotation of the MPMR, providing a slight asymmetry in relation to the contralateral clavicle.

1.2.5. FUNCTION

Its main actions on the arm are medial rotation, powerful adduction, elevation and abduction together with the shoulder. As a secondary function, this muscle elevates the upper ribs, throws and pushes the arm.

1.2.6. MAKING THE FLAP (SURGICAL TECHNIQUE)

Initially, a complete, non-isolated myocutaneous flap was described, which followed the course of the vascular pedicle from the clavicular region to the sternocostal portion of the pectoralis major muscle. In some situations, this flap required a second surgical procedure to section the pedicle. Subsequently, an isolated myocutaneous flap was made, which became popular and is still used today. Some modifications to the original technique have been described in order to adapt the flap to specific defects or to increase its arc of rotation and minimise donor site morbidity. In Brazil, Azevedo's(122) publication stands out. As well as proposing to pass the flap through a subclavicular tunnel, it preserved the clavicular portion of the pectoralis major muscle, which allowed for better function of the ipsolateral arm in movements

against resistance forwards and downwards. The flap can have many variations in technique, such as: flap with two skin islands(123, 124), flap with parasternal skin island over the 3rd intercostal space(125), myofascial flap(123), osteomyocutaneous flap with inclusion of a rib segment(126) and infraclavicular rotation. The latter is a technique that aims to increase the length of the pedicle and, consequently, increase the reach of the flap, with some publications reporting safety and a cosmetic benefit(127).

To summarise, the flap is made by demarcating the size of the skin island, which should be slightly larger than the size of the defect, as there may be retraction of the skin portion after the flap is elevated. The skin island is demarcated in the sternocostal portion of the muscle, between the areola and the sternum, with a lower limit at the upper edge of the seventh rib. The skin island is incised with a cold blade and then with electrocautery up to the pectoralis major muscle fascia. The fascia is then fixed to the skin so as not to damage the perforating vessels when the flap is mobilised. The flap is elevated in the inferior plane of the pectoralis major muscle, which is detached from the costal grill, and its lateral and medial portions are also incised. Between the fourth and sixth intercostal spaces, several perforating vessels from the intercostal branches of the internal thoracic artery are identified, which are cauterised next to the rib cage. From this point, the skin of the flap is perfused by intramuscular anastomoses, located at the level of the 4th rib, between the pectoral branch of the thoracoacromial artery and the intercostal perforating vessels. The main pedicle of the flap is then identified on the underside of the pectoralis major muscle, and the accessory pedicles are also identified as the dissection proceeds superiorly. An auxiliary skin incision can be made on the anterior chest wall from the upper edge of the skin line to the midpoint of the clavicle to improve muscle exposure. An alternative to this approach is to extend the auxiliary incision laterally to the anterior axillary line or to make a subcutaneous tunnel to the clavicular plane, which preserves the integrity of the deltopectoral flap. Once the pectoralis major muscle has been exposed and the vascular pedicles identified, the medial and lateral portions of the muscle that do not contain the pedicle vessels are sectioned under direct vision. The flap is then elevated to the mid-clavicular point and the pedicle is thinned to near its origin in the axillary vessels. Below the pedicle, the lateral pectoral nerve is identified, which should be sectioned to increase the arc of rotation. Care must be taken to avoid traction or twisting that could compromise the arterial irrigation or venous drainage of the flap. The donor area can be closed primarily by detaching the skin flaps and advancing them.

Finally, following the anatomical description of the MPMR, it is clear that it is possible to create an island of skin with a satisfactory area for the reconstruction of large defects based solely on the sternocostal fascicle of the pectoralis major muscle and its main vascular pedicle as the pectoral branch of the thoracoacromial artery. The literature is very rich on this subject, with several studies describing this anatomical characterisation and valuing the flap in cervicofacial reconstructions for its versatility and ability to repair complex defects(128-131).

However, there are few indications for the more cranial reconstructions of the face (forehead, orbit and auricle)(132-135), probably because surgeons have doubts about whether or not they can reach the defect site. Some authors found that there were differences in the origin of the vascular trunk of this flap in relation to the patient's side, being more lateral on the left and more medial on the right(136, 137).

Craniofacial defects and defects in the middle and upper third of the face following extensive tumour resections are one of the most extreme situations for reconstructive surgeons(138). This is due to the anatomical complexity of the structures involved, the three-dimensional configuration of the resulting defect and the great functional and aesthetic impact it has on the patient. The maxilla is the central support structure of the face with great functional and aesthetic importance. It has a three-dimensional configuration in the shape of a hexagon, provides support for the structures of the orbital cone, separates the oral and nasal cavities, forms the basis for dentition and contributes to facial conformation and symmetry. Reconstruction of this segment of the face, for example, becomes imperative and presents varying degrees of complexity depending on the extent of the resection. There are currently a number of treatment options for craniofacial defects and the middle third of the face, ranging from the use of prophetic materials, local flaps, free flaps or a combination of these(139). The use of free flaps is the first choice of services that use this reconstruction technique.

However, as explained above, the use of the microsurgical technique is not yet a reality in many services that treat head and neck cancer, particularly in our country. So could MPMRI also be used for this type of reconstruction? The doubt that hangs over its indication for repairing this type of defect lies, as previously mentioned, in its reach to the higher regions of the face. Even in intraoral defects affecting the hard palate, there may be doubts about the flap's reach in a given case.

Taking into account the different biotypes that exist in the human population, it can be questioned whether the reach of pectoralis major myocutaneous flaps to different cervicofacial anatomical sites is constant, invariable or influenced by individual anthropometric factors. It can also be questioned whether infraclavicular rotation brings benefits in relation to reach, since it is well known that passing the flap under the clavicle is not technically easy; manoeuvres such as elevating the shoulder to increase the subclavicular space and using some lubricant product on the flap, such as sterile liquid Vaseline, to facilitate its passage, may be necessary. In other words, is it possible that for a given individual, the MPMR would be applicable to a specific defect, and in another individual this flap would not be a good option for the same defect? No studies were found in the literature that addressed this question, nor did any explore the determination of the length of the pedicle of the PMMR in order to try to predict its reach.

CHAPTER 2

OBJECTIVES

The objectives of the study are:

- To determine whether infraclavicular rotation provides a significant gain in the reach of the pectoralis major myocutaneous flap to the various sites in the cervicofacial region compared to supraclavicular rotation.

- To determine whether the length of the vascular pedicle and the reach of the pectoralis major myocutaneous flap to the various sites in the cervicofacial region is influenced by the dissection side and anthropometric factors.

CHAPTER 3

MATERIALS AND METHODS

3.1. DELINEATION

Cross-sectional anatomical study.

3.2. CASUISTICS

3.2.1. CADÁVERES

Fifty flaps (25 on the right and 25 on the left) were dissected from 25 adult male cadavers (over 21 years of age) with less than 24 hours since death, which had not been formalised and had not suffered trauma or manipulation of the cervicothoracic region, provided by the University of São Paulo's Death Verification Service (SVO-USP), according to official letter number 041/2009 (Appendix A). Female cadavers were not included in order to better standardise the study, since the breast can hinder the exact positioning of the skin island.

The purpose of initially using cadavers in this thesis was to serve as a basis for conducting a subsequent clinical study. It is therefore imperative that the safety of the procedure is assessed before it is indicated to patients. For example, it would not be ethically possible to test the rotation route, as dissection of the clavicle and extensive manipulation of the flap could lead to comorbidities for the patient and loss of the flap. Similarly, a study should not be carried out on patients without first knowing that at least some anthropometric data had the potential to predict the flap's reach or the length of the pedicle. The results of the cadaver study were also used to calculate the sample size for the clinical study, .

3.2.2. PATIENTS

The sample calculation model used was a hypothesis test for a proportion. The percentage of the flap reaching the orbit via the supraclavicular route in the cadaver study (40%) was used as a reference and the real proportion in the population was set at 15%. A test power of 75% and statistical significance of 5% were adopted, and a sample of 13 male patients was calculated for the surgical procedure and reconstruction with a pectoralis major myocutaneous flap. It was then decided to include 15 patients for a possible loss of 15%. All patients were operated on at one of the Head and Neck Surgery Departments at the ABC Medical School (Padre Anchieta Teaching Hospital or Mário Covas State Hospital).

3.3. ETHICS

This study was authorised and approved by the Research Ethics Committee of the Faculdade de Medicina do ABC, under protocol number 087/2009 (Appendix B) and the Research Ethics Committee of the Faculdade de Medicina da ABC.

University of São Paulo, under protocol 067/2010 (Appendix C). All the patients included agreed to take part in the study and signed an informed consent form (Appendix D).

3.4. POSITIONING AND DATA COLLECTION

Those included in the study were placed in a horizontal dorsal decubitus position with the head in a neutral position and the arms parallel to the body. The following cadaver and patient data was recorded (Annex A and B respectively):

- Demographic data: race (white and non-white) and age;
- Anthropometric data: height, weight, body mass index (BMI), mastoid-furcula

sternal costal distance (MFD), acromiotrochanteric distance (ATD), biacromial distance (BCD) and sternal length (SL), for typological characterisation. The ratio between DMF and CE, between DMF and DAT and between DMF and DBA was also obtained, as shown in Figure 2. The purpose of determining these ratios was to establish relationships between the length of the neck and the thoracic dimensions of the individuals.

- Dissection side: right and left;
- Route of rotation: supra and/or infraclavicular.

Anthropometric parameters such as mastoid-furcula sternal costal distance, acromiotrochanteric distance, biacromial distance and sternal length were measured after fixing the anatomical points with a sterile, disposable 0.3 x 40.0 millimetre (mm) needle and passing the tape measure from one end to the other in a straight line.

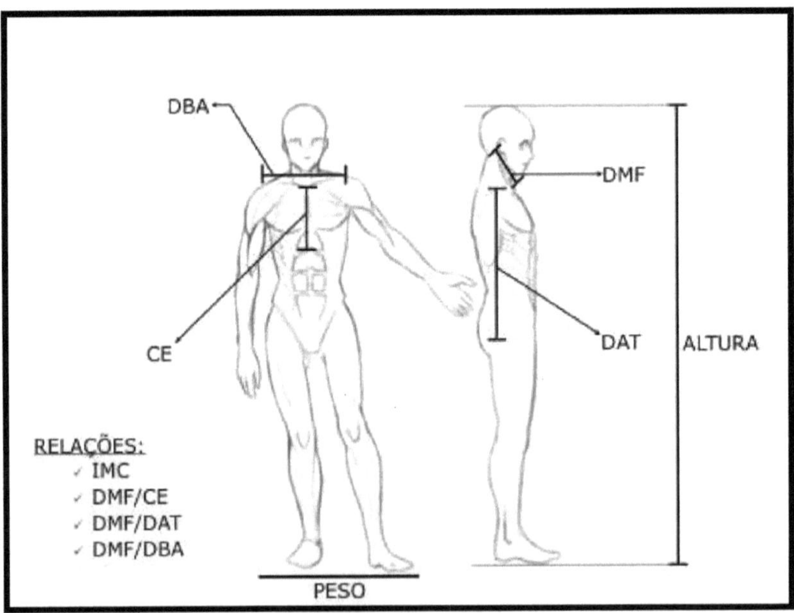

Figure 2: Anthropometric parameters to be measured.

3.5. DISSECTION TECHNIQUE

For each procedure, a standardised 8 cm x 6 cm rectangular skin island was marked out, with its lateral limit on a line parallel to the sagittal plane, starting at the lower edge of the pectoralis major muscle at the level of the 6th intercostal space, next to the upper edge of the 7th rib, and extending 8 cm superiorly, tangential to the medial edge of the ipsilateral nipple. The lower limit of the skin island was obtained through a line 6 cm long perpendicular to the first, drawn over the 6th intercostal space, near the upper edge of the 7th rib. The medial and superior limits were drawn

in the sagittal and axial planes parallel to the other two sides of the rectangle and with the same measurements (Figure 3). This positioning of the skin island was chosen because it includes a second vascular territory of the flap, or caudal vascular territory, which is located between the 4º, 5º and 6º intercostal spaces. The pectoralis major muscle in this region has its irrigation primarily based on several perforating arteries originating in the intercostal branches of the internal thoracic artery. These perforating vessels are located in the intercostal spaces between the sternum and the projection of the nipple over the ribs. In the 4th intercostal space, near the medial edge of the nipple, Rikimaru et al.(140) identified a larger perforating vessel, clinically important for flap perfusion and relatively constant. These two vascular territories communicate with each other through a system of *choke vessels* located at the level of the 4ª costal cartilage. When the pectoralis major muscle is elevated in a caudal-cranial direction and the intercostal perforating arteries have their flow interrupted, the pressure gradient between the cranial and caudal vascular territories is reduced. This allows this system to dilate, communicating the two territories and making the pectoral muscle an axial flap based on the pectoral branch of the thoracoacromial artery with a stable and very reliable vascularisation for the flap skin island. The size of the flap skin island in this study was based on the work of Daniel et al.(141) who studied the dimensions of the tongue using nuclear magnetic resonance. These authors identified an average tongue length of 7.5 ± 0.5 cm and a width of up to 5.1 cm in male patients. Based on these measurements and considering that the tongue is one of the most prevalent sites of head and neck cancer(142), a myocutaneous flap with an 8x6 cm skin island would reconstruct the defect resulting from a total glossectomy, as well as other smaller defects.

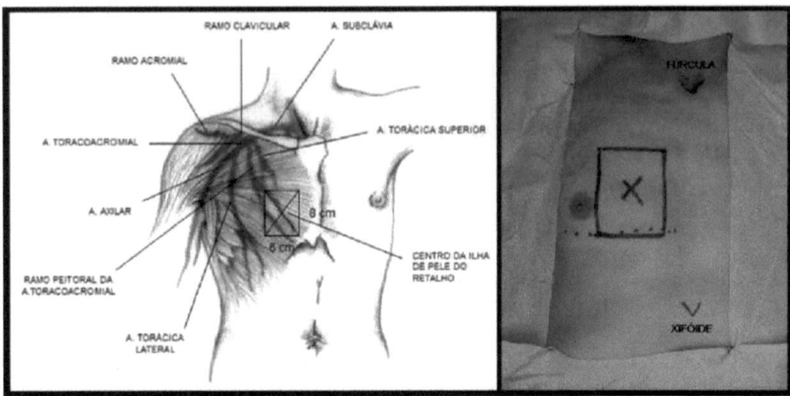

Figure 3: Arterial vascularisation of the pectoralis major muscle. Highlighted is the skin island of the myocutaneous flap that will be pedicled to the pectoral branch of the thoracoacromial artery. On the right (illustration), corresponding diagram of the skin island on the cadaver (photograph).

The flaps were composed of this island of skin, subcutaneous cellular tissue and pectoralis major muscle, with its deep fascia as the last plane of the flap. They were elevated to the clavicle in the usual way and as standardised in the literature(143) without twisting or stretching the pedicle (Figures 4-9). They were based only on the pectoral branch of the thoracoacromial artery, disregarding the lateral and superior thoracic arteries (Figures 10-12). At this point, a malleable tape measure graduated in centimetres according to the Brazilian Association of Technical Standards(144, 145) was used and the length of the vascular pedicle was recorded, from the midpoint of the clavicle at its lower edge to the midpoint of the upper edge of the skin island (Figure 13). A sterilised, malleable tape measure of the same model as the one used on the cadavers was used on the patients. The position of the emergence of the pectoral branch of the thoracoacromial artery in relation to the mid-clavicular line was also noted on the cadavers and patients, classifying the pedicles into three types: type A - when the emergence of the pedicle of the PMR is more than two centimetres medial to the mid-clavicular line; type B - when it is up to two centimetres medial or lateral to the mid-clavicular line; type C - when it is more than two centimetres lateral to the mid-clavicular line. This classification is illustrated in Figure 14.

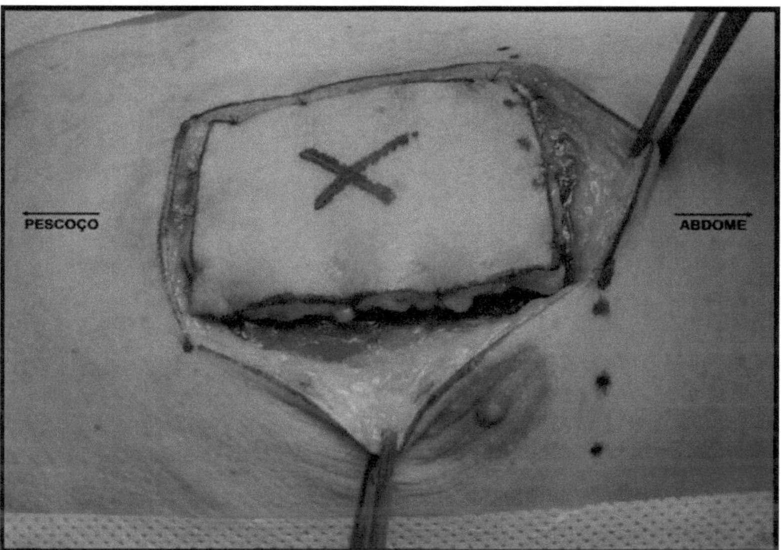

Figure 4: Beginning of the dissection of the flap made up of skin, subcutaneous cellular tissue and the pectoralis major muscle; the skin island is fixed to the muscle plane with stitches so that the flap can be transposed in its entirety.

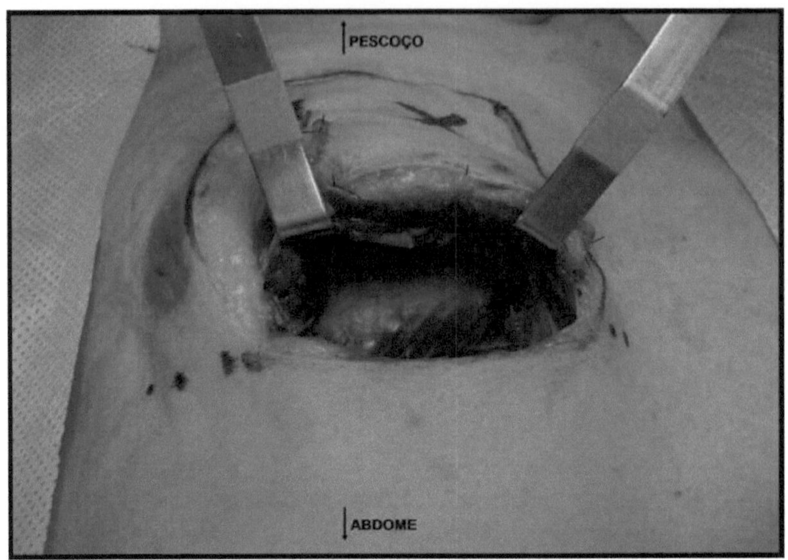

Figure 5: Lower limit of the dissection: the deep fascia of the pectoralis major muscle.

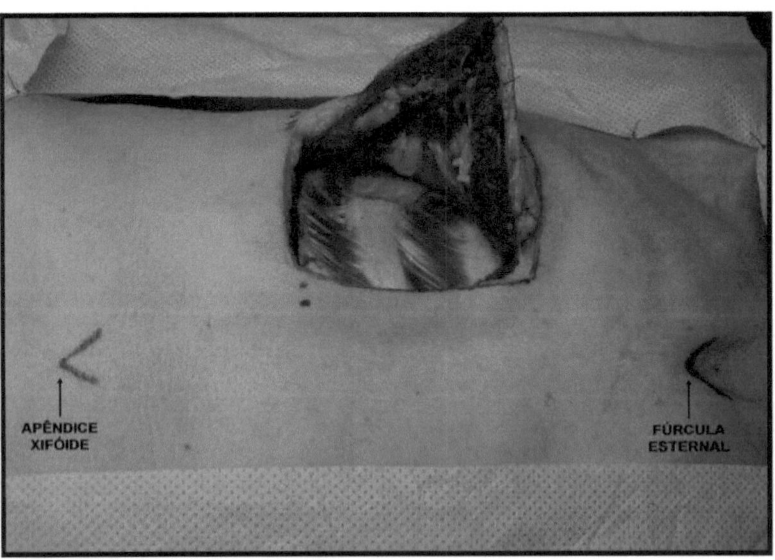

Figure 6: Medial section of the flap.

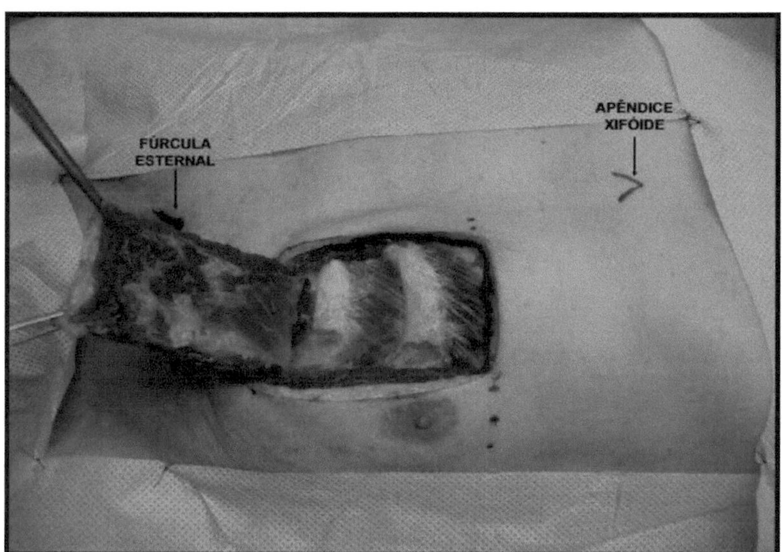

Figure 7. Lateral section of the flap and start of its rotation.

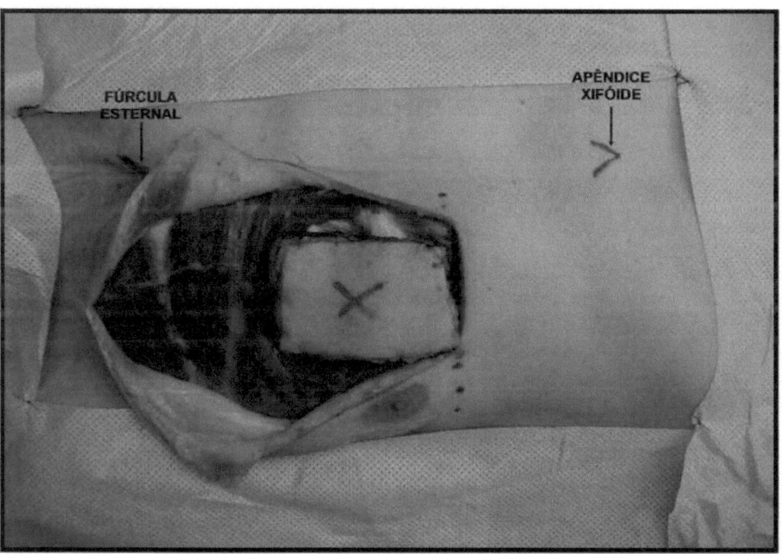

Figure 8. Upper extension of the incision from the midpoint of the upper portion of the skin island to the clavicular midpoint, isolating the pectoralis major muscle.

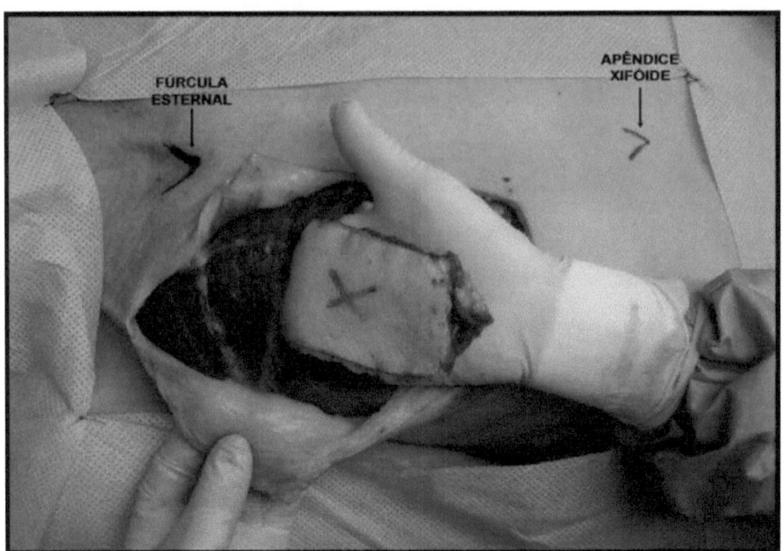

Figure 9. Blunt dissection between the deep fascia of the pectoralis major muscle superiorly and the costal gradient inferiorly.

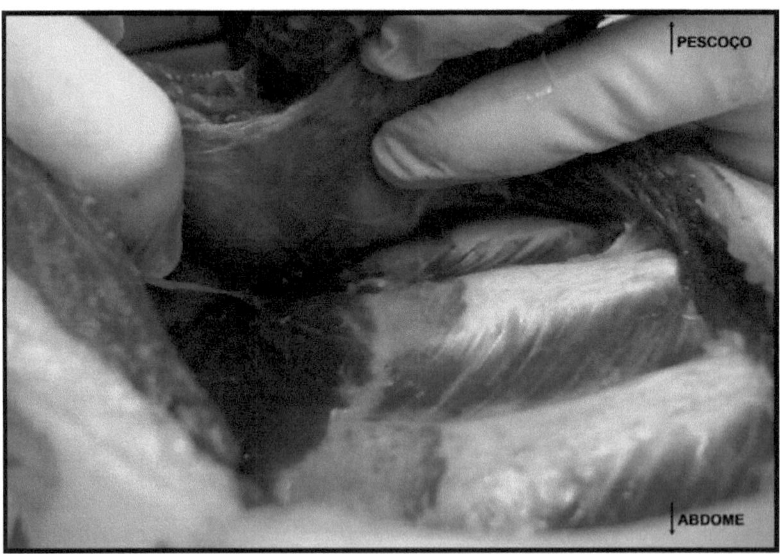

Figure 10. Identification of the vascular pedicle, based on the pectoral branch of the thoracoacromial artery (arrow).

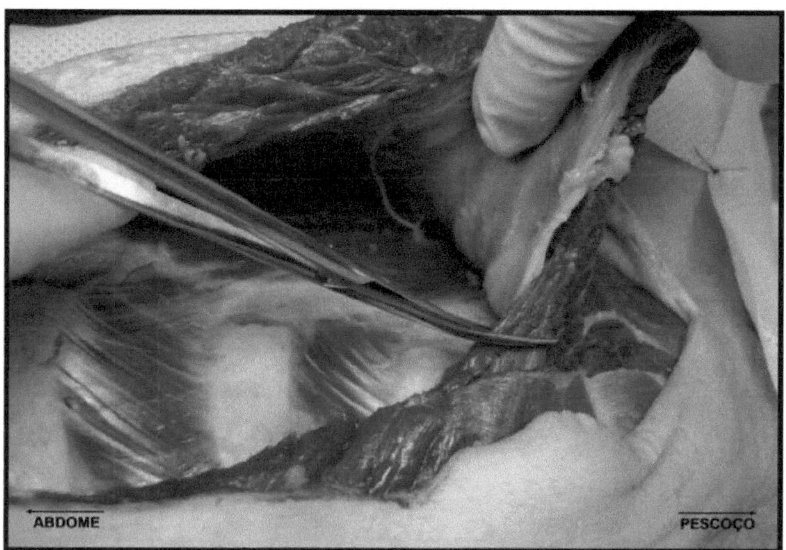

Figure 11. With the pedicle identified, the pectoralis major muscle is sectioned medially to the lower edge of the clavicle.

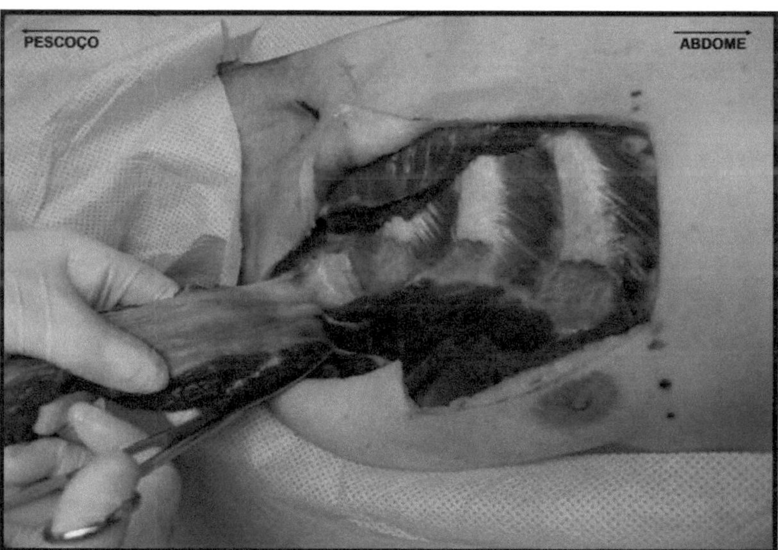

Figure 12. After the medial section, the pectoralis major muscle is sectioned laterally up to the lower edge of the clavicle, taking care to keep the vascular pedicle intact.

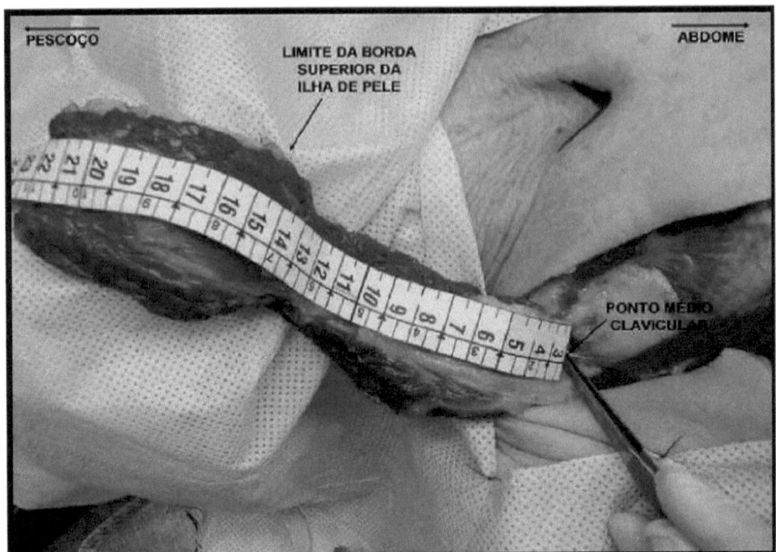

Figure 13. Supraclavicular rotation of the flap and measurement of its pedicle: from the clavicular midpoint at its lower edge to the level of the midpoint of the upper edge of the skin island.

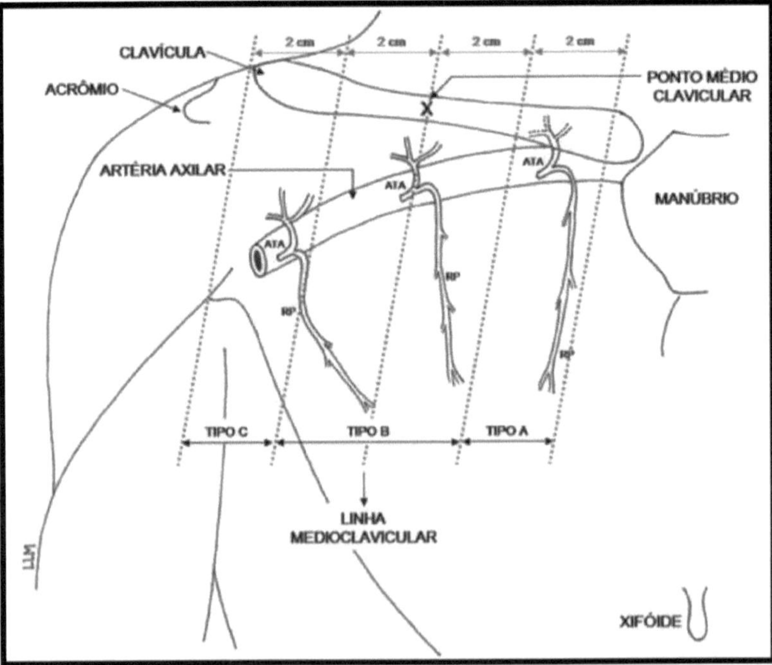

Figure 14. Types of emergence of the pectoral branch of the thoracoacromial artery. Type A: when medial beyond 2 cm from the medioclavicular line. Type B: when distant medially or laterally from the medioclavicular line by up to 2 cm. Type C: when lateral beyond 2 cm

from the medioclavicular line. Legend: ATA - thoracoacromial artery; RP - pectoral branch of the thoracoacromial artery(146).

The flap was then rotated supraclavicularly to the cervicofacial region, without twisting or traction of the vascular pedicle, and the range of the flap centre (determined by crossing the two medians of the right angles of the rectangular skin island as shown in Figure 3) was analysed for the orbit, external auditory canal, angle of the mandible, chin and laryngeal prominence of the thyroid cartilage(147). The scope for these sites of the cervicofacial surface anatomy in the cadaver aims to determine the possibility of reconstruction for the following clinical situations, maintaining the integrity of the pedicle, without torsion or tension: orbit - defects resulting from enlarged maxillectomies with exenteration; external auditory canal - defects of the parotid region and ear; angle of the mandible - defects of the retromolar area and oropharynx; chin - defects of the tongue and floor; laryngeal prominence of the thyroid cartilage - defects of the hypopharynx (Figure 15)(148). After this step, the flap was transposed via the infraclavicular route, only in the cadavers, and the same reaches were tested to assess whether this manoeuvre determines an effective gain in flap reach. The length of the pedicle was measured again after infraclavicular rotation.

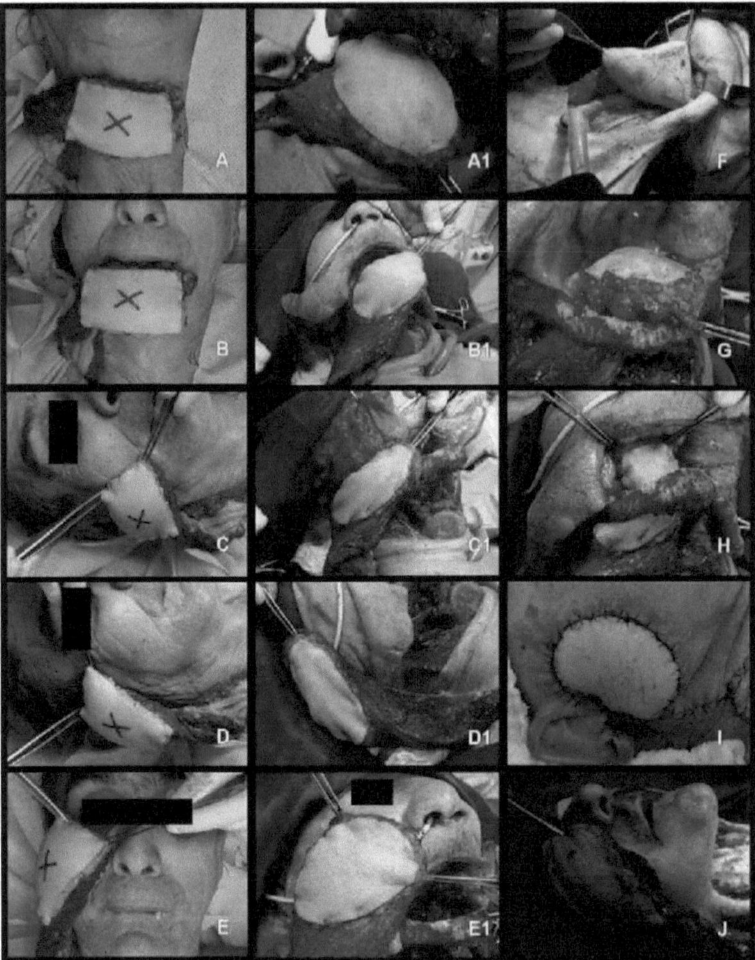

Figure 15. Supraclavicular rotation of the MPMRI and its reach to the cervicofacial region *in the* cadaver (left column) and the respective correspondences *in vivo* (centre column): A and A1 - laryngeal prominence of the thyroid cartilage; B and B1 - chin; C and C1 - angle of the mandible; D and D1 - external auditory canal; E and E1 - attempt to reach the orbit. Right column: clinical situations showing the reconstruction of defects corresponding to the anatomical sites mentioned: F - hypopharynx; G - oral tongue; H - retromolar area and oropharynx; I - parotid region; J - upper cervicofacial region and orbit. Note: The clinical cases illustrated in the centre and right columns were not part of this protocol and were photographed only to demonstrate the correspondence of the surface anatomy sites tested in the study and the defects corresponding to these sites.

At the end of the dissection, the flap was resutured to the donor area in the cadaver and in the patients the subsequent surgical steps were re-established, i.e. the flap was transposed and sutured to the surgical defect and the donor area was closed. In the case of the cadavers, all the incisions and sutures were made in topographical regions that preserved the external appearance of the cadavers (Figure 16), following SVO-USP standards. In the clinical trial, i.e. with the patients, there were no manoeuvres that altered the therapeutic approach or put their integrity at risk. Also in the patients, after an 8x6cm square flap had been elevated, corrections were made to the shape of this island of skin when necessary, using dehydermisation to adapt it to the defect.

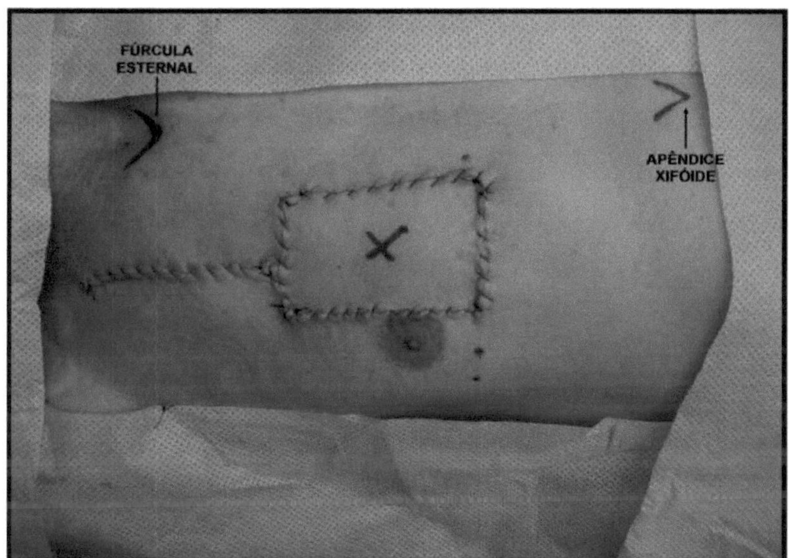

Figure 16. Final aspect of the dissection after suturing the skin island to the donor area.

3.6. EVALUATION OF RESULTS AND STATISTICAL ANALYSIS

The length of the pedicle and the length of the flap for the various sites in the cervicofacial region were compared with the anthropometric data previously described and with the dissection side of all the cases studied. As mentioned above, the flap length for these sites was compared between the supraclavicular and infraclavicular rotation routes for the cadavers only.

The values obtained from the study of each quantitative variable were organised and described using the mean and standard deviation, and absolute and relative frequencies were used for the qualitative variables. The categorical variables dissection side and flap reach had the following possibilities: dissection side (right or left); flap reach to a particular region (yes or no).

SPSS® version 17.0 (SPSS® Inc; Ilinois, USA) was used for statistical analysis. The distributions were defined as parametric or non-parametric using the Kolmogorov-Smirnov test. Student's f-test was used to compare the means of two sample populations and the chi-squared test was used to compare the frequency of a phenomenon between groups of qualitative variables. To check for correlation between two quantitative variables, the Pearson and Spearman correlation tests were used to assess parametric and non-parametric variables, respectively. In the multivariate analysis, the linear regression model was used to create a risk prediction equation.

The risk of committing a type I error of less than 5% was considered in all analyses ($p < 0.05$).

CHAPTER 4

RESULTS

4.1. ANALYSING THE CORPSE

4.1.1. CLINICAL CHARACTERISTICS AND DESCRIPTIVE DATA

As previously described, the study consisted of 25 adult male cadavers who had their PMR dissected bilaterally and transposed to the cervicofacial region. The descriptive data of the cadavers included in the study, their demographic and anthropometric measurements, as well as the length of the vascular pedicle, its position in relation to the medioclavicular line and the reach of the flap to the various cervicofacial sites are shown in Table 1. The complete table with all the data collected can be found in Appendix C.

Table 1. Descriptive data of the cadavers.

FEATURES	RESULT
Age (years)* Ethnicity**	66,28 ± 9,58 (48-87)
White	36 (72%)
Non-white	14 (28%)
Weight (kg)*	72,80 ± 9,83 (50-93)
Height (m)*	1,75 ±0,07 (1,64-1,90)
BMI (kg/m^2)*	23,83 ±3,04 (15,43-29,41)
DMF (cm)*	18,67 ± 1,47 (16,0-22,0)
EC (cm)*	20,52 ± 1,76 (16,0-24,0)
DAT (cm)*	59,43 ± 4,32 (47,0-72,0)
DBA (cm)*	32,20 ± 2,32 (28,0-37,0)
DMF/CE*	0,91 ±0,09 (0,75-1,19)
DMF/DAT*	0,32 ± 0,02 (0,26-0,37)
DMF/DBA*	0,58 ± 0,06 (0,47-0,73)
Pedicle length (cm)*	
Supraclavicular	17,67 ±2,24 (12,0-22,0)
Infraclavicular	18,28 ±2,24 (13,0-22,0)
Pedicle position**	
Right side	B: 25(100%)
Left side	B: 23(92%); C: 2(8%)
Retail reach by route***	
Supraclavicular	
Orbit	20 (40%)
External auditory canal	50 (100%)
Jaw angle	50 (100%)
Mento	50(100%)

Laryngeal prominence of the thyroid cartilage	50 (100%)
Infraclavicular	
Orbit	22 (44%)
External auditory canal	50 (100%)
Jaw angle	50 (100%)
Mento	50 (100%)
Laryngeal prominence of the thyroid cartilage	50 (100%)

* Mean ± Standard deviation (minimum-maximum)
** Position in relation to type A, B and C
*** Absolute numbers (percentage)

4.1.2. RETAIL RANGE

As for the reach, the analysis was only carried out for the orbit, since in all the cases analysed the other reaches tested were reached (thyroid cartilage, chin, mandibular angle and external auditory canal) in both rotations. The univariate analysis showed that there was a statistically significant difference in the reach of the flap to the orbit by supraclavicular rotation in individuals with a greater acromiotrochanteric distance - ATD (p= 0,008 - Student's t-test), greater biacromial distance - DBA (p= 0.024 - Student's t-test) and a lower ratio of mastoid to sternal furcula distance - DMF/DAT (p= 0.005 - Student's t-test). It was also observed that cadavers whose flaps reached the orbit were statistically heavier (p=0.036 - Student's t-test). The other comparisons of flap reach with anthropometric data showed no statistically significant differences. The full results are detailed in Tables 2 and 3.

Table 2. Analysis of the flap's reach to the orbit by supraclavicular rotation in relation to the dissection side in cadavers.

FEATURES	REACH TO ORBIT*		SIGNIFICANCE
	YES	NO	
QUALITATIVE"			
Dissection side			
Law	10	15	n-d nnn
Left	10	15	p- I ,uuu

LEGEND:
■ chi-squared test
* Absolute numbers (qualitative variables); mean ± standard deviation (quantitative variables)

Table 3. Analysis of the flap's reach to the orbit by supraclavicular rotation in relation to anthropometric variables in cadavers.

FEATURES	REACH TO ORBIT*		SIGNIFICANCE
	YES	NO	
QUANTITATIVE⁰			
Weight (kg)	76,35 ± 9,57	70,43 ± 9,43	p=0,036**

Height (m)	1,76 ±0,08	1,74 ±0,06	p=0,311
BMI (kg/m²)	24,62 ± 2,71	23,29 ±3,17	p=0,132
DMF (cm)	18,55 ± 1,39	18,75 ± 1,53	p=0,642
EC (cm)	20,7 ± 1,49	20,4 ± 1,94	p=0,561
DAT (cm)	61,37 ±4,38	58,13 ±3,82	p=0,008**
DBA (cm)	33,10 ±2,22	31,6 ±2,22	p=0,024**
DMF/CE	0,89 ± 0,08	0,92 ±0,1	p=0,341
DMF/D AT	0,30 ± 0,02	0,32 ± 0,02	p=0,005**
DMF/DBA	0,56 ± 0,05	0,59 ± 0,06	p=0,053

LEGEND:
□ Student's t-test
* Absolute numbers (qualitative variables); mean ± standard deviation (quantitative variables)
* * p: statistical significance level less than 0.05

Infraclavicular rotation of the flap did not affect the reach to the orbit according to the univariate analysis (p=0.839 - chi-squared test). Studying each case individually, when infraclavicular rotation was performed, there was a gain in reach to the orbital region in two cases, which represented approximately 9% (2/22 cases) of the flaps that reached the orbit and 4% of the entire series. In one of the dissections, however, the flap failed to reach the orbit due to infraclavicular rotation, while in the same case supraclavicular rotation provided adequate reach (Table 4). The fact that infraclavicular rotation did not provide a gain in the reach of the PMFRI to the cervico-facial region of the cadavers led us not to test this route of PMFRI rotation in the clinical study, described below

Table 4. Analysis of the flap's reach into the orbit in relation to the route of rotation.

CASES	REACH TO ORBIT**		SIGNIFICANCE AND TEST USED
	SUPRA-CLAVICULAR ROTATION	INFRA-CLAVICULAR ROTATION	
Case 4D	Yes	Yes	
Case 4E	Yes	Yes	
Case 6D	Yes	Yes	
Case 6E	Yes	No	
Case 7D	Yes	Yes	
Case 7E	Yes	Yes	
Case 8D	Yes	Yes	
Case12D	Yes	Yes	
Case12E	Yes	Yes	
Case13E	Yes	Yes	
Case16D	Yes	Yes	
Case 16E	Yes	Yes	**p=0,839**
Case18D	Yes	Yes	**(chi-squared)**

Case18E	Yes	Yes
Case19D	Yes	Yes
Case 19E	Yes	Yes
Case 20D	Yes	Yes
Case 20E	Yes	Yes
Case 22D	Yes	Yes
Case 22E	Yes	Yes
Case 23D	No	Yes
Case 23E	No	Yes
TOTAL***	20/22 (90,90%)	21/22 (95,45%)

1 Case (dissection side)
2 * Including cases in which the orbit was reached by at least one of the rotation routes.
3 ** Absolute numbers and (percentages)

4.1.3. VASCULAR PEDICLE LENGTH

The length of the flap's vascular pedicle ranged from 12 cm to 22 cm, with a mean of 17.67 ± 2.24 cm for supraclavicular rotation (Figure 17). In infraclavicular rotation, the average length of the vascular pedicle was 18.28 cm with a standard deviation of ± 2.24 cm (minimum of 13 cm and maximum of 22 cm), i.e. there was a gain of 0.61 cm in the average length of the pedicle when compared to the average for supraclavicular rotation. There was also a statistical difference with a positive correlation between the two measurements ($r = 0.765$; $p<0.0001$ - Pearson's correlation test) but, as shown above, although there was an increase in the length of the pedicle in the infraclavicular passage, there was no gain in the reach of the flap compared to supraclavicular rotation.

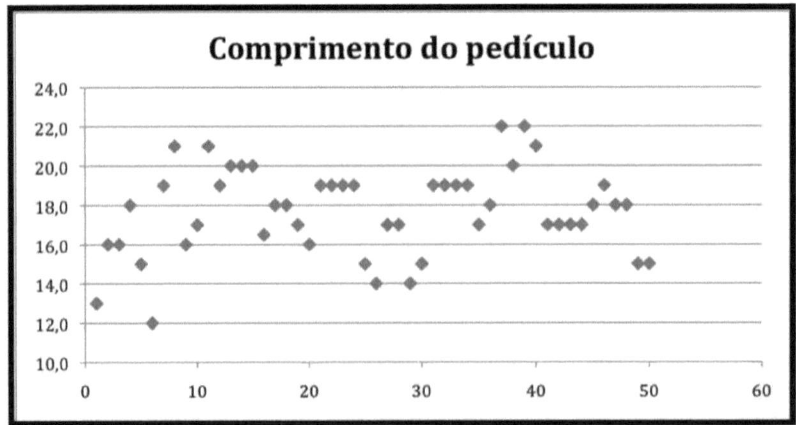

Figure 17. Dispersion of individual pedicle length values (in centimetres) in cadavers by

supraclavicular rotation.

In the univariate analysis, there was a positive and statistically significant correlation between the length of the pedicle per supraclavicular rotation and the biacromial distance - DBA (r= 0.311; p= 0.028 - Pearson's correlation); negative correlation and also significant with the ratio between the mastoid-sternal furcula distance and the biacromial distance - DMF/DBA (r= -0.362; p= 0.010 - Pearson's correlation) and with the ratio between the mastoid-sternal furcula distance and the acromiotrochanteric distance - DMF/DAT (r= -0.403; p= 0.004 - Pearson's correlation). The other comparisons and correlations relating to pedicle length showed no statistically significant differences. The full results are detailed in Tables 5 and 6.

Table 5. Analysis of pedicle length by supraclavicular rotation in relation to anthropometric variables and in relation to the dissection side in cadavers.

FEATURES	PEDICLE LENGTH*	SIGNIFICANCE
COMPARISON'		
Dissection side		
Law	17,72 ±2,35	p=0,876
Left	17,62 ±2,16	

LEGEND:
■ Student's t-test
* Mean ± Standard deviation for comparisons

Table 6. Analysis of vascular pedicle length by supraclavicular rotation in relation to anthropometric variables in cadavers.

FEATURES	PEDICLE LENGTH*	SIGNIFICANCE
CORRELATIONS⁰		
Weight (kg)	r=-0,114	p=0,431
Height (m)	r= 0,103	p=0,478
BMI (kg/m²)	r=-0,169	p=0,241
DMF (cm)	r=-0,232	p=0,105
EC (cm)	r=-0,162	p=0,260
DAT (cm)	r= 0,152	p=0,292
DBA (cm)	r= 0,311	p=0,028 **
DMF/CE	r=-0,033	p=0,820
DMF/DAT	r=-0,362	p=0,010**
DMF/DBA	r=-0,403	p=0,004 **

LEGEND:
* Pearson's correlation test
* Mean ± Standard deviation for comparisons and Person's correlation coefficient ("r") for correlations
* * p: level of statistical significance less than 0.05

Once the presence of anthropometric factors associated with the length of the vascular pedicle of the PMR in cadavers had been proven, a basis was obtained for carrying out the clinical study, the results of which are presented below.

4.2. ANALYSING PATIENTS

4.2.1. CLINICAL CHARACTERISTICS AND DESCRIPTIVE DATA

As previously described, the study consisted of 15 adult male patients who had their MPMRs dissected and transposed to the cervicofacial region only by supraclavicular rotation during the surgical procedure. The calculation of this sample was based on the result of reaching the orbit in the cadaver study and is shown in Appendix D. In 8 patients the flap was made on the right side and in the remaining cases on the left. The descriptive data of the patients included in the study, their demographic and anthropometric measurements, the length of the vascular pedicle, its position according to the proposed typological classification (types A, B and C) and the flap's reach to the various cervicofacial sites are shown in Table 7. The complete table with all the data collected can be found in Appendix E.

Table 7. Descriptive data from the clinical study.

FEATURES	RESULT
Age (years)* Ethnicity**	60,67 ±9,49 (48-81)
White	6(40%)
Non-white	9(60%)
Weight (kg)*	62,73 ± 15,18 (40-91)
Height (m)*	1,70 ±0,05 (1,60-1,80)
BMI (kg/m²)*	21,40 ±4,42 (14,20-28,07)
DMF (cm)*	18,23 ± 1,09 (16,00-20,00)
EC (cm)*	18,23 ± 1,09 (16,00-20,00)
DAT (cm)*	57,16 ±3,65 (46,00-61,00)
DBA (cm)*	33,53 ± 2,78 (29,00-38,00)
DMF/CE*	0,84 ± 0,09 (0,73-0,95)
DMF/DAT*	0,31 ± 0,01 (0,28-0,35)
DMF/DBA*	0,54 ± 0,04 (0,47-0,62)
Pedicle length (cm)*	16,03 ± 1,35 (13,50-18,00)
Pedicle position**	

Right side	B: 8(100%)
Left side	B: 7(100%)
Reach of the flap by supraclavicular route* **	
Orbit	2 (13,30%)
External auditory canal	15 (100%)
Jaw angle	15 (100%)
Mento	15(100%)
Laryngeal prominence of the thyroid cartilage	15(100%)

* Mean ± Standard deviation (minimum-maximum)

* Position in relation to type A, B and C

* Absolute numbers (percentage)

4.2.2. RETAIL RANGE

In terms of reach, only the orbit was analysed, since in all the cases analysed the other reaches tested were achieved (thyroid cartilage, chin, mandibular angle and external auditory canal). Infraclavicular rotation was not assessed as there was already evidence in the cadaver study that this route of rotation does not contribute to the gain in terms of MPMRI range for the cervicofacial sites to be reconstructed.

Of the 15 patients included in the clinical study, only two cases reached the orbit (13.3%). It was therefore decided not to carry out the statistical analysis, since the small number of outcomes would make the statistical power of the tests very low.

3.6.1. VASCULAR PEDICLE LENGTH

The length of the vascular pedicle of the live flap ranged from 13.5 cm to 18 cm, with an average of 16.03 ± 1.35 cm (Figure 18).

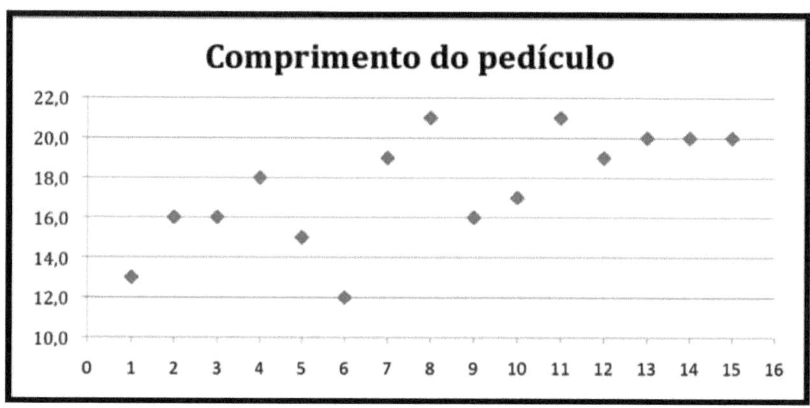

Figure 18. Dispersion of individual pedicle length values (in centimetres) in the clinical study.

In the univariate analysis, there was a positive and statistically significant correlation between the length of the pedicle and the length of the sternum - CE (r= 0.722; p= 0.002 - Sperman's correlation) and a negative and also significant correlation with the ratio between the mastoid-sternal furcula distance and the length of the sternum - DMF/CE (r= -0.587; p= 0.021 - Sperman's correlation). The other comparisons and correlations relating to pedicle length showed no statistically significant differences. The full results are detailed in Table 8.

Table 8. Analysis of vascular pedicle length in relation to anthropometric variables in the clinical study.

FEATURES	PEDICLE LENGTH*	SIGNIFICANCE
Age	r= 0,136	p=0,630
Weight (kg)	r= 0,368	p=0,177
Height (m)	r= 0,514	p=0,050
BMI (kg/m²)	r= 0,295	p=0,286
DMF (cm)	r= 0,057	p=0,839
EC (cm)	r= 0,722	p=0,002**
DAT (cm)	r= 0,271	p=0,329
DBA (cm)	r= 0,438	p=0,103
DMF/CE	r=-0,587	p=0,021**
DMF/DAT	r=-0,142	p=0,612
DMF/DBA	r=-0,474	p=0,074

LEGEND:
1 Sperman's correlation coefficient ("r")
2 * p: level of statistical significance less than 0.05

With the results obtained from the univariate statistical analysis, the variables with p<0.20 were subjected to multivariate analysis using a linear regression model, with the aim of establishing the equation for predicting the length of the vascular pedicle. The variables included were: weight, height, CE, DBA, DMF/CE and DMF/DBA. The only variable capable of determining the length of the vascular pedicle of the PMR was the length of the sternum (p=0.004 - linear regression).

On the basis of this regression data, an equation was established to determine the length of the vascular pedicle of the RMPM (COMP) based on the length of the sternum, as shown below:

$$\textbf{COMP = 2.54 + 0.64 X CE}$$

According to this model, the higher the EC value, the greater the length of the vascular pedicle.

CHAPTER 5

DISCUSSION

The tools that head and neck surgeons have in the reconstructive field are constantly being improved, both in terms of new techniques and the refinement of those already in use. Often, anatomical studies initially answer certain doubts about the applicability of these technological advances, which can then be transposed into clinical practice. This is why we were encouraged to carry out this study, as there has been no anatomical study in the literature on cadavers or in clinical practice to date that has attempted to objectively relate the length of the RMPM and its reach into the cervicofacial region to individual anthropometric characteristics, the side of dissection and the route of rotation.

Currently, the incidence of head and neck cancers has increased along with the constant need to perfect reconstruction techniques with the aim of preserving function, cosmetic effect and, above all, cure. In recent decades, various types of reconstruction have been used, such as free grafts, prostheses, local flaps, pedicled flaps and microsurgical free flaps(149-151), as discussed at length in the Introduction. However, perhaps none of these other techniques is as important and versatile as the pectoralis major myocutaneous flap, first described by Stephan Ariyan over thirty years ago and the subject of many discussions and anatomical studies, often referred to as the workhorse of reconstructive surgery in the head and neck (110).

This technique has several qualities: it provides adequate thickness, sufficient skin coverage, a reliable vascular pedicle, a good arc of rotation, resistance to surgical infection, good coverage for the cervical vessels with obliteration of the dead space, a simple technique, primary closure of the donor area in the chest wall and the ability to reconstruct most cervicofacial defects in a single surgical time(152, 153). In addition to these advantages, it also has low complication rates even when performed after radiotherapy and allows high doses of adjuvant ionising radiation to be used in the tumour resection area without major additional complications(100, 154). It can also be used as a therapeutic option in the treatment of post-operative complications, such as fistulas or tissue necrosis, or in elderly patients and those with comorbidities such as vasculopathy, diabetes, hypertension or heart disease, in which there are clinical limitations to the use of free flaps. Over the years, it has proved to be a reliable flap even in the most difficult cases(155, 156).

Despite the aesthetic and functional superiority of microsurgical reconstructions over pedicled flaps, PMR also has good results and, according to some authors, lower surgical and hospital costs, achieving acceptable rehabilitation with low loss rates and easy clinical and post-operative follow-up, and is considered simpler to manage when compared to microsurgical flaps(157). On the other hand, there are authors who argue that there is no difference in the various socio-psycho-economic aspects of the two types of reconstruction(18), and others who recognise the better applicability of both flaps in the different indications for reconstruction(158).

Despite the versatility of the MPMRI, as initially described and proven in clinical practice in various reconstructed areas such as the hypopharynx(159), oral cavity, oropharynx(160) and parotid region(161, 162), few studies have described the MPMRI for reconstruction of more cranial facial defects such as the orbit(7), probably due to the surgeon's doubts about the possibility of the flap reaching the defect region. In situations involving complex defects of the upper part of the mouth, including the hard palate and sometimes the skin of the maxillary region, there may also be doubts about the reach of the MPMRI. In one of his early works, Ariyan describes the flap he developed for various regions, including the orbit(110). Among the most commonly used flaps for this type of reconstruction is the McGregor frontal flap, first described in 1963, which offers a large amount of skin, a constant vascular pedicle and a good arc of rotation(39, 163). Today, its indication is considered an exception due to its aesthetic disadvantage compared to that provided by microsurgical flaps(164).

The first important piece of anatomical data confirmed during this study was the main vascularisation of the flap by the pectoral branch of the thoracoacromial artery, which was clearly isolated in all cases without difficulty. As shown in several previous studies, its vascular supply area is 13x20 cm between the third and fourth ribs, up to 24 cm from the medioclavicular line(114, 165, 166). In the individual analysis, two cases were found in cadavers in which there was a lateralisation of the pedicle exit in relation to the axillary artery, only on the left side of the dissection. This finding is corroborated by the study by Nakajima et al.(136) who identified anatomical differences in the origin of the arterial pedicle between the right and left sides, with it being more lateral on the left and more medial on the right. Park et al.(137), in another anatomical study on the vascular anatomy of the pectoralis major flap, classified the origin of the pectoral branch of the thoracoacromial artery into three groups: type I - the origin of the pectoral branch occurs directly from the trunk of the thoracoacromial artery (78.6% of cases, 29 cases on the right and 26 on the left); type II - the origin of the pectoral branch occurs from the medial pedicle of the thoracoacromial artery (15.7% of cases, four on the right and seven on the left); type III - the origin of the pectoral branch occurs from the lateral pedicle of the thoracoacromial artery (5.7% of cases, one on the right and three on the left). In this same study, it was observed that the thoracoacromial artery originated in all cases from the axillary artery, and that its point of origin was around 2 to 3 cm inferior to the clavicle. In relation to the clavicle, the origin of the thoracoacromial artery on the right side was lateral to the medioclavicular line in 100% of cases, while on the left it was located medial to it in 86% of cases. This study therefore shows a clear variation between the right and left sides in the origin of the vascular pedicle of the MPMR, based on the medioclavicular line. The existence of these aforementioned anatomical variations justifies the finding, in two of our cases, of a more lateral pedicle located on the left. In one of these cases of a more lateral pedicle, the PMR reached the orbit only by supraclavicular rotation.

The loss of reach to the orbit due to infraclavicular rotation, which occurred in this specific case, is explained by the fact that rotation through the infraclavicular passage only takes place through the clavicular midpoint. Since the coracoid process of the scapula is located at the same height as the exit of this more lateral pedicle, which prevents the flap from passing through, the useful length of the pedicle is lost so that it can be rotated through the clavicular midpoint. In this same situation, supraclavicular rotation can be carried out laterally to the clavicular midpoint and does not result in a reduction in the useful length of the MPMR pedicle (Figure 19)(148). In the other case in which a more lateral pedicle was observed, the two rotations did not reach the orbit, but during the passage of the flap under the clavicle there was also a reduction in the useful length of the vascular pedicle.

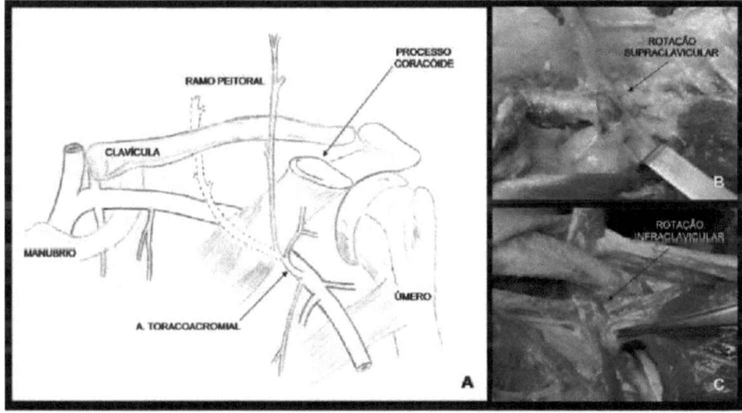

Figura 19. Demonstration of the loss of range in infraclavicular rotation of the MPMR in individuals with the thoracoacromial artery in a lateral position. Schematic representation (A); supraclavicular (B) and infraclavicular (C) rotation in the cadaver.

As explained in the Materials and Methods section, we classified the origin of the flap's main pedicle into three types: type A - when the pedicle emerges more than two centimetres medially to the medioclavicular line; type B - when the pedicle emerges up to two centimetres medially or laterally to the medioclavicular line; type C - when the pedicle emerges more than two centimetres laterally to the medioclavicular line. Figure 14 illustrates this classification.

As a result, we found that on the right side (25 dissected flaps), all the pedicles were type B and that on the left (25 dissected flaps) we observed 23 type B pedicles (92%) and two type C pedicles (8%). No type A pedicles were identified in the cadavers. In the patients, all the vascular pedicles were type B. We can state that in pedicles with an emergence greater than 2 cm lateral to the mid-clavicular line (type C), there is a clear reduction in the flap's reach by infraclavicular rotation when compared to supraclavicular rotation because, as explained above, the pedicle must initially describe a path towards the midpoint of the clavicle and then be transposed underneath it, which results in a loss of its useful length (146). This anatomical data shows that there are differences in the position of the pedicle between the right and left sides. A possible explanation for this difference lies in the fact that the subclavian artery (which continues as the axillary artery) originates directly from the aortic arch on the left and on the right it originates more laterally from the innominate artery (brachiocephalic arterial trunk). If we analyse the anatomical diagrams (Figure 20), we can see that, in relation to the midline, the origin of the left subclavian artery is more lateralised when compared to the origin of the right subclavian artery, which may explain the occurrence of a more lateralised PMR vascular pedicle in some cases on the left, both in our series and in those of other authors cited here.

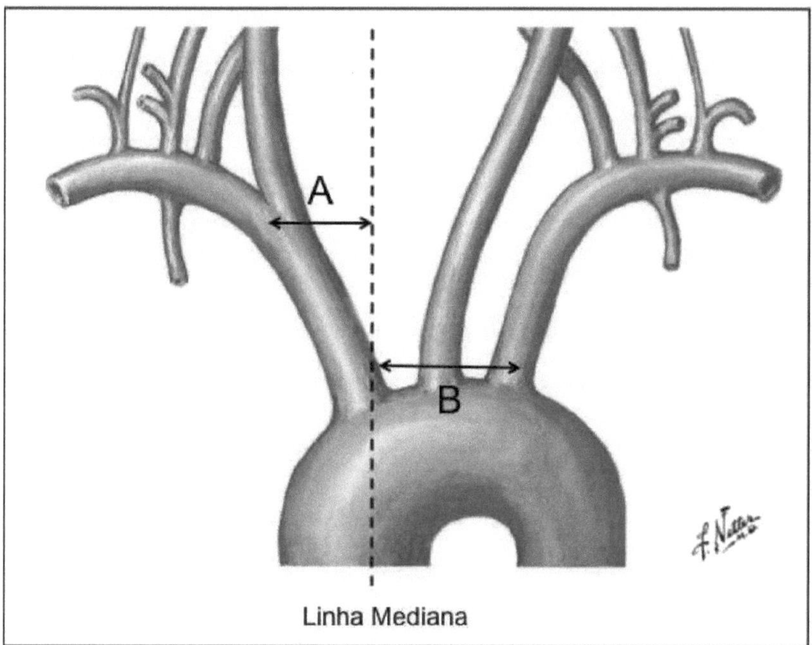

Figure 20. Anatomical representation of the more lateralised origin (B) in relation to the midline of the left subclavian artery, when compared to the origin of the right subclavian artery (A) - adapted with permission.

In head and neck reconstructive surgery, it should often be borne in mind that the search for the best option for reconstruction should be the one with the lowest degree of complexity, the shortest surgical time and the aim of correcting the defect definitively. This justifies the choice of most surgeons to use the pectoralis major flap by supraclavicular rotation and the importance of establishing simple parameters that can be transposed to clinical practice, ensuring greater applicability in the surgical routine, as this study aims to do.

With regard to the route of rotation, the data in the literature consulted is conflicting as to which would be the safest and most beneficial route. According to a study by Kerawala et al.(167), although no statistically significant difference was found between the complications of flaps transposed over and under the clavicle, the casuistry of these authors is small and in the individual analysis of each case, there is an increase of almost 50% in complications in cases of infraclavicular passage, such as partial or total loss and infection. Vartanian et al.(68), in different population samples of supraclavicular and infraclavicular passages, observed greater individual complications in cases of supraclavicular rotation. In the present study, despite the fact that no vascular lesions were observed in the infraclavicular passage in any of the flaps made in the cadavers, rotation under the clavicle did not bring statistically significant benefits in relation to the reach of the flap to the orbit, while for the other regions the reach is easily obtained in the traditional way.

With regard to the length of the vascular pedicle, this study found an average length of 17.67 ± 2.24cm and 16.03 ± 1.35cm in the patients, both by supraclavicular rotation, with the measurement being taken from the clavicular midpoint to the upper edge of the skin island, as standardised. This length provided an adequate arc of rotation to reconstruct the various anatomical sites studied, which correspond to most of the defects to be reconstructed. In 100% of cases, the flap was able to reconstruct the defect generated by the surgical treatment of tumours of the oral cavity, oropharynx, hypopharynx, parotid region and skin of the cervical region, without putting the pedicle at risk or increasing surgical time with the infraclavicular passage. Despite various studies on this flap, no reference was found in the literature consulted regarding the length of the pedicle of the MPMR. Following evidence in the cadaver study that there is an association between the length of the vascular pedicle and individual anthropometric factors, these relationships were analysed in the 15 patients included in the study, and it was concluded that the length of the sternum is the only factor determining the length of the vascular pedicle of the PMVR. The equation **COMP = 2.54 + 0.64 X CE,** obtained by linear regression, allows the length of the pedicle of the PMR to be determined preoperatively, approximately and with a small margin of error, with a skin island of identical dimensions and positioning to the one used in this study. Although the length of the pedicle did not influence the extent of the PMMR in this study, prior determination of the length of the vascular pedicle can provide more appropriate planning for reconstruction in specific clinical situations. In this work, for example, we studied the reach from the centre of the skin island to a fixed point on the surface anatomy. In certain clinical situations, it may be more important to determine whether the distal end of the skin island can reach the distal end of the defect. Thus, by previously determining the length of the pedicle of an 8 cm x 6 cm quadrangular flap with its lower limit at the upper edge of the 7ª rib, it will theoretically be possible to adequately plan the dimensions, shape and positioning of the MPMRI skin island that is to be used in a particular circumstance, in order to guarantee a greater chance of the flap reaching the defect adequately and, consequently, a successful reconstruction. As explained by Tincani et al.(93), it is possible to extend the skin island to the level of the rectus abdominis muscle in order to increase the flap's reach to the more cranial regions of the face. In these situations, prior knowledge of the length of the vascular pedicle of the MPMR, as standardised in this study, can help determine the necessary length of this skin area with random vascularisation, reducing the risk of distal necrosis of the flap.

Regarding the reach of the MPMRI, it was shown that this flap has a constant reach for most topographies of the head and neck, with the exception of the orbit, which was reached in 40% of cases in cadavers and only 13% of patients, which shows that the MPMRI should not be considered as the first option for reconstruction of this topography. However, as discussed above, based on the size of the defect to be reconstructed, with prior knowledge of the length of the pedicle and the size of the skin island to be used, one can theoretically programme the reconstruction of regions neighbouring the orbit, such as the skin of the cheek, for example.

This study has therefore provided new data that could be useful for clinical practice. The results obtained suggest that by analysing the patient's anthropometry, it may be possible to predict the length of the PMR pedicle and indirectly its reach, especially for more cranial defects. In addition, it was possible to objectively determine that infraclavicular rotation does not benefit the reach of the MPMRI to the head and neck region, and even reduces this reach in some situations, so its use is not justified.

CHAPTER 6

CONCLUSIONS

From the above we conclude that:

- Infraclavicular rotation of the pectoralis major myocutaneous flap does not increase the flap's reach to the cervicofacial region compared to supraclavicular rotation;

- The length of the vascular pedicle and the reach of the pectoralis major myocutaneous flap are not influenced by the dissection side and the only anthropometric variable that can estimate the length of the pedicle is the length of the sternum.

CHAPTER 7

ANNEXES

7.1. ANNEX A: Death Verification Service Study Protocol.

LARGER BREAST PROTOCOL 8 cm X 6 cm
N⁰.: SVO.: SIDE:
RACE:_____ AGE:_______WEIGHT:____ HEIGHT:_______BMD: _____
EC: _____
DAT: ____
DBA: ____
DMF/CE:______
DMF/DAT : ____
DMF/DBA : ____

4 Pedicle identification:
()YES( )NO
5 Pedicle length:
a) Supraclavicular rotation: _______ b) Infraclavicular rotation: _________
6 Pedicle injury in infraclavicular rotation:
()YES( )NO
7 Reach of the retail centre:
a) Thyroid cartilage furcula
a.1.) Supraclavicular rotation: () YES () NO
a.2.) Infraclavicular rotation: () YES () NO
b) Mento
b.1.) Supraclavicular rotation: () YES () NO
b.2.) Infraclavicular rotation: () YES () NO
c) Jaw angle
c.1.) Supraclavicular rotation: () YES () NO
c.2.) Infraclavicular rotation: () YES () NO
d) External auditory canal
d.1.) Supraclavicular rotation: () YES () NO
d.2.) Infraclavicular rotation: () YES () NO
e) Orbit
f) 1.) Supraclavicular rotation: () YES () NO
g) 9 \ Rntacăn infrcmlaviri ilar (\ RIM (\ MĂA

7.2. ANNEX B: Clinical Study Protocol (Patients)

LARGER BREAST PROTOCOL 8 cm X 6 cm - LIVE
N⁰.: _____ SIDE:_____
RACE:_____ AGE: ______
WEIGHT:___ HEIGHT: ______
DMF: ____
EC: _____
DAT: ____
DBA: ____
DMF/CE:___
DMF/DAT : ____
DMF/DBA : ____

8 Pedicle identification:
()YES() NO
9 Pedicle length:

a) Supraclavicular rotation: _______

10 Reach of the retail centre:

h) Thyroid cartilage furcula

()YES() NO

i) Mento

()YES() NO

j) Jaw angle

()YES() NO

k) External auditory canal

()YES() NO

l) Orbit

( ) YES ( ) NO

7.3. ANNEX C: Cadaver data

SVO nº	RAÇA (B=1;NB=2)	IDADE	PESO	ALTURA	IMC	DMF	CE	DAT	DBA	DMF/CE	DMF/DAT	DMF/DBA	ID PED (S=1;N=0)	LD DISSEC (D=1;E=2)	Comp supra	Comp Infra	orbita Supra (N=0;S=1)	Orb Infra(N=0;S=1)
Caso 1D	1	80	84	1,72	28,39	17,5	22,0	63,0	30,0	0,80	0,28	0,58	1	1	13,0	14,0	0	0
Caso 1E	1	80	84	1,72	28,39	18,0	22,0	61,0	30,0	0,82	0,30	0,60	1	2	16,0	16,0	0	0
Caso 2D	1	75	70	1,64	26,03	19,0	22,0	63,0	28,0	0,86	0,30	0,68	1	1	16,0	17,0	0	0
Caso 2E	1	75	70	1,64	26,03	18,0	22,0	62,0	28,0	0,82	0,29	0,64	1	2	18,0	19,0	0	0
Caso 3D	1	54	60	1,70	20,76	18,0	24,0	58,0	29,0	0,75	0,31	0,62	1	1	15,0	16,0	0	0
Caso 3E	1	54	60	1,70	20,76	19,0	24,0	58,0	29,0	0,79	0,33	0,66	1	2	12,0	14,0	0	0
Caso 4D	1	65	75	1,66	27,22	19,0	20,0	54,0	29,0	0,95	0,35	0,66	1	1	19,0	16,0	1	1
Caso 4E	1	65	75	1,66	27,22	18,0	20,0	57,0	29,0	0,90	0,32	0,62	1	2	21,0	21,0	1	1
Caso 5D	2	58	70	1,70	24,22	18,0	20,0	57,0	29,0	0,90	0,32	0,62	1	1	16,0	17,0	0	0
Caso 5E	2	58	70	1,70	24,22	18,0	20,0	56,0	29,0	0,90	0,32	0,62	1	2	17,0	18,0	0	0
Caso 6D	2	53	60	1,70	20,76	17,0	19,0	57,5	34,0	0,89	0,30	0,50	1	1	21,0	19,0	1	1
Caso 6E	2	53	60	1,70	20,76	16,0	19,0	56,0	34,0	0,84	0,29	0,47	0	2	19,0	17,0	1	0
Caso 7D	1	62	90	1,90	24,93	19,0	24,0	72,0	37,0	0,79	0,26	0,51	1	1	20,0	22,0	1	1
Caso 7E	1	62	90	1,90	24,93	19,0	24,0	70,0	37,0	0,79	0,27	0,51	1	2	20,0	22,0	1	1
Caso 8D	1	53	74	1,80	22,84	20,0	20,0	60,0	34,0	1,00	0,33	0,59	1	1	20,0	21,0	1	1
Caso 8E	1	53	74	1,80	22,84	20,0	20,0	60,0	34,0	1,00	0,33	0,59	0	2	16,5	13,0	0	0
Caso 9D	1	65	65	1,70	22,49	19,0	19,0	61,0	34,0	1,00	0,31	0,56	1	1	18,0	20,0	0	0
Caso 9E	1	65	65	1,70	22,49	19,0	19,0	62,0	34,0	1,00	0,31	0,56	1	2	18,0	20,0	0	0
Caso 10D	2	63	78	1,80	24,07	21,0	21,0	62,0	31,0	1,00	0,34	0,68	1	1	17,0	19,0	0	0
Caso 10E	2	63	78	1,80	24,07	20,0	21,0	61,0	31,0	0,95	0,33	0,65	1	2	16,0	18,0	0	0
Caso 11D	1	62	76	1,70	26,30	19,0	20,0	56,0	34,0	0,95	0,34	0,56	1	1	19,0	13,0	0	0
Caso 11E	1	62	76	1,70	26,30	18,0	20,0	57,0	34,0	0,90	0,32	0,53	1	2	19,0	17,0	0	0
Caso 12D	1	67	85	1,80	26,23	19,0	19,0	58,0	31,0	1,00	0,33	0,61	1	1	19,0	19,0	1	1
Caso 12E	1	67	85	1,80	26,23	18,0	19,0	59,0	31,0	0,95	0,31	0,58	1	2	19,0	19,0	1	1
Caso 13D	1	70	93	1,90	25,76	22,0	22,0	64,0	34,0	1,00	0,34	0,65	1	1	15,0	15,0	0	0
Caso 13E	1	70	93	1,90	25,76	22,0	22,0	65,0	34,0	1,00	0,34	0,65	1	2	14,0	14,0	1	1
Caso 14D	1	48	70	1,70	24,22	19,0	20,0	58,0	31,0	0,95	0,33	0,61	1	1	17,0	17,0	0	0
Caso 14E	1	48	70	1,70	24,22	19,0	20,0	57,0	31,0	0,95	0,33	0,61	1	2	17,0	19,0	0	0
Caso 15D	1	72	70	1,70	24,22	16,0	18,0	49,0	32,0	0,89	0,33	0,50	1	1	14,0	17,0	0	0
Caso 15E	1	72	70	1,70	24,22	17,0	18,0	47,0	32,0	0,94	0,36	0,53	1	2	15,0	17,0	0	0
Caso 16D	2	72	75	1,70	25,95	19,0	20,0	64,0	34,0	0,95	0,30	0,56	1	1	19,0	20,0	1	1
Caso 16E	2	72	75	1,70	25,95	19,0	20,0	64,0	34,0	0,95	0,30	0,56	1	2	19,0	20,0	1	1
Caso 17D	1	66	60	1,80	18,52	20,0	22,0	30,0	33,0	0,91	0,36	0,61	1	1	19,0	20,0	0	0
Caso 17E	1	65	60	1,80	18,52	19,0	22,0	56,0	33,0	0,86	0,34	0,58	1	2	19,0	20,0	0	0
Caso 18D	1	55	70	1,70	24,22	17,0	21,0	59,0	33,0	0,81	0,29	0,52	1	1	17,0	17,0	1	1
Caso 18E	1	55	70	1,70	24,22	17,0	21,0	60,0	33,0	0,81	0,28	0,52	1	2	18,0	17,0	1	1
Caso 19D	2	75	70	1,80	21,60	18,0	21,0	62,0	31,0	0,86	0,29	0,58	1	1	22,0	22,0	1	1
Caso 19E	2	75	70	1,80	21,60	19,0	21,0	61,0	31,0	0,90	0,31	0,61	1	2	20,0	20,0	1	1
Caso 20D	2	77	70	1,80	21,60	17,0	22,0	62,0	33,0	0,77	0,27	0,52	1	1	22,0	22,0	1	1
Caso 20E	2	77	70	1,80	21,60	18,0	22,0	61,0	33,0	0,82	0,30	0,55	1	2	21,0	21,0	1	1
Caso 21D	1	60	80	1,80	24,69	18,0	20,0	60,0	35,0	0,90	0,30	0,51	1	1	17,0	19,0	0	0
Caso 21E	1	60	80	1,80	24,69	18,0	20,0	59,0	35,0	0,90	0,31	0,51	1	2	17,0	19,0	0	0
Caso 22D	1	77	85	1,70	29,41	20,0	20,0	63,0	35,0	1,00	0,32	0,57	1	1	17,0	19,0	1	1
Caso 22E	1	77	85	1,70	29,41	20,0	20,0	63,0	35,0	1,00	0,32	0,57	1	2	17,0	19,0	1	1
Caso 23D	1	71	50	1,80	15,43	19,0	16,0	55,0	34,0	1,19	0,35	0,56	1	1	18,0	19,0	0	1
Caso 23E	1	71	50	1,80	15,43	19,0	16,0	57,0	34,0	1,19	0,33	0,56	1	2	19,0	20,0	0	1
Caso 24D	2	67	70	1,70	24,22	16,0	19,0	55,0	30,0	0,84	0,29	0,53	1	1	18,0	19,0	0	0
Caso 24E	2	67	70	1,70	24,22	16,0	19,0	55,0	30,0	0,84	0,29	0,53	1	2	18,0	19,0	0	0
Caso 25D	1	71	70	1,80	21,60	22,0	22,0	60,0	30,0	1,00	0,37	0,73	1	1	15,0	17,0	0	0
Caso 25E	1	71	70	1,80	21,60	21,0	22,0	59,0	30,0	0,95	0,36	0,70	1	2	15,0	17,0	0	0

7.4. ANNEX D: Sample calculation for the clinical study

Values calculated with input data

Proportion of the population: **15%**
Suggested proportion: **40%**
Level of significance: **5%**
Test power: **75%**
Hypothesis test: **one-tailed**
Calculated sample size: **13**
For other values of the significance level and power of the test we have:

Level of meaning	Test power	Sample size
5%	65%	10
5%	70%	11
5%	S0%	16
5%	85%	19
5%	90%	24
5%	95%	31
0.1%	75%	33
1%	75%	22
10%	75%	10

7.5. ANNEX E: Clinical study data

N	IDADE	PESO	ALTURA	IMC	LADO RETALHO (1=D, 2=E)	ALCANCE RETALHO ÓRBITA (1=SIM, 0=NÃO)	COMPRIMENTO PEDÍCULO	CE	DBA
1	74	50,0	1,6	19,1	2	1	16,1	21,0	33,0
2	70	45,0	1,7	16,1	1	0	16,0	21,0	33,0
3	65	90,9	1,8	28,7	2	0	16,5	21,5	34,5
4	71	86,0	1,7	28,7	1	0	17,0	22,0	38,0
5	57	77,6	1,8	24,0	1	0	18,0	24,5	36,0
6	59	64,0	1,8	20,7	2	0	18,0	24,5	31,5
7	81	80,0	1,7	27,7	2	0	17,0	20,5	31,0
8	59	40,0	1,7	14,2	1	0	13,5	20,0	30,0
9	51	54,0	1,8	17,6	1	0	17,0	23,0	36,0
10	48	54,3	1,7	19,0	1	0	17,0	23,0	38,0
11	52	61,2	1,8	20,0	2	0	16,0	20,0	36,0
12	59	56,0	1,7	19,8	2	1	18,0	21,5	33,0
13	55	66,0	1,7	23,1	1	0	14,5	20,5	32,0
14	54	50,0	1,6	19,3	1	0	15,0	22,0	29,0
15	63	49,7	1,7	18,0	2	0	16,0	22,0	29,0

N	DAT D	DAT E	DMF D	E	DMFD/CE	DMFE/CE	DMFE/DBA	DMFD/DATD	DMFE/DATE
1	47,0	46,0	15,5	16,0	0,74	0,76	0,48	0,33	0,35
2	57,0	56,5	20,0	20,0	0,95	0,95	0,61	0,35	0,35
3	62,5	61,0	19,0	19,0	0,88	0,88	0,55	0,30	0,31
4	55,0	55,5	18,0	19,0	0,82	0,86	0,50	0,33	0,34
5	61,0	61,0	20,0	20,0	0,82	0,82	0,56	0,33	0,33
6	60,0	59,0	17,5	18,0	0,71	0,73	0,57	0,29	0,31
7	60,0	60,0	18,0	18,0	0,88	0,58	0,30	0,30	0,30
8	54,5	55,5	17,5	17,0	0,88	0,85	0,57	0,32	0,31
9	57,0	56,0	19,0	18,5	0,83	0,80	0,51	0,33	0,33
10	56,0	57,0	18,0	18,5	0,78	0,80	0,49	0,32	0,32
11	57,0	57,0	19,0	19,0	0,95	0,95	0,53	0,33	0,33
12	57,5	58,0	17,0	16,5	0,79	0,77	0,50	0,30	0,28
13	58,0	59,0	18,0	18,5	0,88	0,90	0,58	0,31	0,31
14	59,0	59,0	18,0	18,0	0,82	0,82	0,62	0,31	0,31
15	61,0	62,0	19,0	19,0	0,86	0,86	0,66	0,31	0,31

CHAPTER 8

BIBLIOGRAPHICAL REFERENCES

1. Juri J, Juri C, Cerisola J. Contribution to Converse's flap for nasal reconstruction. Plastic and reconstructive surgery. 1982;69(4):697-702.

2. Rabson JA, Hurwitz DJ, Futrell JW. The cutaneous blood supply of the neck: relevance to incision planning and surgical reconstruction. British journal of plastic surgery. 1985;38(2):208-19.

3. Freeman JL, Walker EP, Wilson JS, Shaw HJ. The vascular anatomy of the pectoralis major myocutaneous flap. Br J Plast Surg. 1981 ;34(1):3-10.

4. Shah JP. Reconstructive surgery. In: Kowalski LP, editor. Head and Neck Surgery. 1 ed. Rio de Janeiro: Revinter; 2000. p. 559-605.

5. McGregor IA. A "defensive" approach to the island pectoralis major myocutaneous flap. Br J Plast Surg. 1981;34(4):435-7.

6. Bakamjian V, Hoffmeister FS. Reconstructive surgery in management of tumours of head and neck. N Y State J Med. 1963;63:301-11.

7. Ariyan S. The pectoralis major for single-stage reconstruction of the difficult wounds of the orbit and pharyngoesophagus. Plast Reconstr Surg. 1983;72(4):468-77.

8. Weiglein AH, Haas F, Pierer G. Anatomic basis of the lower trapezius musculocutaneous flap. Surg Radiol Anat. 1996;18(4):257-61.

9. Tan Q, Zhou HR, Wang SQ, Zheng DF, Xu P, Wu J, et al. Aesthetic effect of wound repair with flaps. Zhonghua Shao Shang Za Zhi. 2012;28(4):248-52.

10. Trojanowski P, Andrzejczak A, Trojanowska A, Olszanski W, Klatka J. Importance of donor site vascular imaging in free fibula flap reconstruction. Otolaryngol PoL 2012;66(4 Suppl):40-4.

11. Klein MB, Donelan MB, Spence RJ. Reconstructive surgery. J Burn Care Res. 2007;28(4):602-6.

12. Hurvitz KA, Kobayashi M, Evans GR. Current options in head and neck reconstruction. Plast Reconstr Surg. 2006;118(5):122e-33e.

13. Ghali S, Knox KR, Boutros S, Thorne CH, McCarthy JG. The incidence of late cephalohematoma following craniofacial surgery. Plast Reconstr Surg. 2007; 120(4): 1004-8.

14. Sugg KB, Cederna PS, Brown DL. The V-Y advancement flap is equivalent to the Mustarde flap for ectropion prevention in the reconstruction of moderate-size lid-cheek junction defects. Plast Reconstr Surg. 2013;131(1):28e-36e.

15. Kendler M, Averbeck M, Wetzig T. Reconstruction of nasal defects with forehead flaps in patients older than 75 years of age. J Eur Acad Dermatol Venereol. 2013.

16. Konofaos P, Hammond S, Ver Halen JP, Samant S. Reconstructive techniques in transoral robotic surgery for head and neck cancer: a north american survey. Plast Reconstr Surg. 2013;131(2):188e-97e.

17. Kilinc H, Geyik Y, Aytekin AH. Double-skin paddled superficial temporofascial flap for the reconstruction of full-thickness cheek defect. J Craniofac Surg. 2013;24(1):e92-5.

18. Smeele LE, Goldstein D, Tsai V, Gullane PJ, Neligan P, Brown DH, et al. Morbidity and cost differences between free flap reconstruction and pedicled flap reconstruction in oral and oropharyngeal cancer: Matched control study. J Otolaryngol. 2006;35(2): 102-7.

19. Wookey H. The surgical treatment of carcinoma of the pharynx and upper oesophagus. Surg Gynecol Obstet 1942;1(499):75.

20. Whitaker IS, Karoo RO, Spyrou G, Fenton OM. The birth of plastic surgery: the story of nasal reconstruction from the Edwin Smith Papyrus to the twenty-first century. Plast Reconstr Surg. 2007;120(1):327-36.

21. Sorta-Bilajac I, Muzur A. The nose between ethics and aesthetics: Sushruta's legacy. Otolaryngol Head Neck Surg. 2007;137(5):707-10.

22. Sankaranarayanan R. Oral cancer in India: an epidemiologic and clinicai review. Oral Surg Oral Med Oral PathoL 1990;69(3):325-30.

23. Sedwick JD, Graham V, Tolan CJ, Sykes JM, Terkonda RP. The full-thickness forehead flap for complex nasal defects: a preliminary study. Otolaryngol Head Neck Surg.

2005;132(3):381-6.

24. Menick FJ. A 10-year experience in nasal reconstruction with the three-stage forehead flap. Plast Reconstr Surg. 2002; 109(6): 1839-55; discussion 56- 61.

25. Furlan S, Mazzola RF. Alessandra Benedetti, a fifteenth century anatomist and surgeon: his role in the history of nasal reconstruction. Plast Reconstr Surg. 1995;96(3):739-43.

26. Li QF, Xie F, Gu B, Zheng D, Lei H, Liu K, et al. Nasal reconstruction using a split forehead flap. Plast Reconstr Surg. 2006; 118(7): 1543-50.

27. Tansini I. Sopra il mio nuovo processo di amputazione delia mamaella per cancre. Goz Med Ital 1906;4:57.

28. Zevallos JP, Urken ML. Reverse-flow scapular osteocutaneous flap for head and neck reconstruction. Head Neck. 2012.

29. Posnick JC, McCraw JB, Magee W, Jr. Use of a latissimus dorsi myocutaneous flap for closure of an orocutaneous fistula of the cheek. J Oral Maxillofac Surg. 1988;46(3):224-8.

30. McCraw JB, Penix JO, Baker JW. Repair of major defects of the chest wall and spine with the latissimus dorsi myocutaneous flap. Plast Reconstr Surg. 1978;62(2): 197-206.

31. Ferbeyre-Binelfa L. Lattissimus dorsi myocutaneous flap in head and neck surgery. Cir Clr. 2010;78(6):7.

32. Kettel K. Surgical treatment of peripheral facial palsy in closed head injuries. Nord Med. 1949;41(8):347-9.

33. Kirschbaum S. Mentosternal contracture; preferred treatment by acromial (in charretera) flap. Plast Reconstr Surg Transplant Buli. 1958;21(2):131-8.

34. Pallua N, Magnus Noah E. The tunneled supraclavicular island flap: an optimised technique for head and neck reconstruction. Plast Reconstr Surg. 2000;105(3):842-51; discussion 52-4.

35. Lamberty BG. The supra-clavicular axial patterned flap. Br J Plast Surg. 1979;32(3):207-12.

36. Di Benedetto G, Aquinati A, Pierangeli M, Scalise A, Bertani A. From the "charretera" to the supraclavicular fascial island flap: revisitation and further evolution of a controversial flap. Plast Reconstr Surg. 2005;115(1):70-6.

37. Alves HRNI, L.C.; Besteiro, J.M.; Cernea, C.; Gemperli, R.; Brandão, L.G.; Ferreira, M.C. Supraclavicular flap: a new reconstructive option after resection of extensive skin tumours in head and neck surgery. Rev Bras Cir Cabeça Pescoço. 2010;40(3):114-9.

38. McGregor JA, Reid WH. The use of the temporal flap in the primary repair of full-thickness defects of the cheek. Plast Reconstr Surg. 1966;38(1):1- 9.

39. McGregor IA. The Temporal Flap in Intra-Oral Cancer: Its Use in Repairing the Post-Excisional Defect. Br J Plast Surg. 1963;16:318-35.

40. McGregor IA. The pursuit of function and cosmesis in managing oral cancer. Br J PlastSurg. 1993;46(1):22-31.

41. Antunes AAAAP. Reconstruction of the exenteric orbital cavity: free skin graft or temporofrontal flap? Rev Cir Traumatol Buco- Maxilo-Fac. 2006;6(1):9-14.

42. Lore JM. General purpose flaps. In: Lore JM, editor. An atlas of nead and necksurgery. 3rd ed. ed. Philadelphia, P.A.: Saunders Company, W.B.; 1998. p. 364-9.

43. Vanni CMRSP, F.R.; Kanda, J.L. Temporofrontal Pedicle Flap in Head and Neck Surgery. Arq Bras Cien Sau. 2010;32(2):99-102.

44. Bakamjian VY. A Two-Stage Method for Pharyngoesophageal Reconstruction with a Primary Pectoral Skin Flap. Plast Reconstr Surg. 1965;36:173-84.

45. Saint-Cyr M, Schaverien MV, Rohrich RJ. Perforator flaps: history, controversies, physiology, anatomy, and use in reconstruction. Plast Reconstr Surg. 2009; 123(4): 132e-45e.

46. Morain WD. Cari Manchot, plastic surgery's missed opportunity. Med Herit. 1985; 1(3): 174-80.

47. Andrews BT, McCulloch TM, Funk GF, Graham SM, Hoffman HT. Deltopectoral flap revisited in the microvascular era: a single-institution 10-year experience. Ann Otol Rhinol Laryngol. 2006; 115(1):35-40.

48. Mutter TD. Case of Deformed Leg, from Unsuccessfully Treated Fracture: Cured by Operation. Prov Med J Retrosp Med Sei. 1842;4(94):285-7.

49. Zovickian A. Pharyngeal fistulas: repair and prevention using mastoid- occiput based shoulder flaps. Plast Reconstr Surg (1946). 1957;19(5):355-72.

50. Conley J. Use of composite flaps containing bone for major repairs in the head and neck. Plast Reconstr Surg. 1972;49(5):522-6.

51. Demergasso F, Piazza MV. Trapezius myocutaneous flap in reconstructive surgery for head and neck cancer: an original technique. Am J Surg. 1979;138(4):533-6.

52. Baek SM, Biller HF, Krespi YP, Lawson W. The lower trapezius island myocutaneous flap. Ann Plast Surg. 1980;5(2):108-14.

53. Conley JJ. The prevention of carotid artery haemorrhage by the use of rotating tissue flaps. Surgery. 1953;34(2): 186-94.

54. Conley JJ, Clairmont AA. Practical suggestions in facial plastic surgery-- how i do it. "Threading" augmentation for facial wrinkles. Laryngoscope. 1976;86(12): 1886-90.

55. Ugurlu K, Ozcelik D, Huthut I, Yildiz K, Kilinc L, Bas L. Extended vertical trapezius myocutaneous flap in head and neck reconstruction as a salvage procedure. Plast Reconstr Surg. 2004,114(2):339-50.

56. Mathes DW, Thornton JF, Rohrich RJ. Management of posterior trunk defects. Plast Reconstr Surg. 2006;118(3):73e-83e.

57. Hagan KM, S.J. Trapezius muscle and musculocutaneous flaps. Grabb's Encyclopaedia of flaps. 2nd ed. ed: Lippincott-Ravens Pub; 1998. p. 461-6.

58. Tan KC, Tan BK. Extended lower trapezius island myocutaneous flap: a fasciomyocutaneous flap based on the dorsal scapular artery. Plast Reconstr Surg. 2000; 105(5): 1758-63.

59. Urken ML, Naidu RK, Lawson W, Biller HF. The lower trapezius island musculocutaneous flap revisited. Report of 45 cases and a unifying concept of the vascular supply. Arch Otolaryngol Head Neck Surg. 1991;117(5):502-11.

60. Fox JW, Edgerton MT. The fan flap: an adjunct to ear reconstruction. Plast Reconstr

Surg. 1976;58(6):663-7.

61. Panje WR, Morris MR. The temporoparietal phasia flap in head and neck reconstruction. Ear Nose Throat J. 1991 ;70(5):311-7.

62. Pinto FR, de Magalhaes RP, Capelli Fde A, Brandao LG, Kanda JL. Pedicled temporoparietal galeal flap for reconstruction of intraoral defects. Ann Otol Rhinol LaryngoL 2008; 117(8):581-6.

63. Pinto F, Magalhaes R, Durazzo M, Brandao L, Rodrigues Jr AJ. Galeal flap based on superficial temporal vessels for oral cavity and pharynx reconstruction--an anatomical study. Clinics (Sao Paulo). 2008;63(1):97-102.

64. Nayak VK, Deschler DG. Pedicled temporoparietal fascial flap reconstruction of select intraoral defects. Laryngoscope. 2004; 114(9): 1545-8.

65. Petruzzelli GJ, Brockenbrough JM, Vandevender D, Creech SD. The influence of reconstructive modality on cost of care in head and neck oncologic surgery. Archives of otolaryngology--head & neck surgery. 2002;128(12):1377- 80.

66. Milenovic A, Virag M, Uglesic V, Aljinovic-Ratkovic N. The pectoralis major flap in head and neck reconstruction: first 500 patients. J Craniomaxillofac Surg. 2006;34(6):340-3.

67. El-Marakby HH. The reliability of pectoralis major myocutaneous flap in head and neck reconstruction. J Egypt Natl Canc Inst. 2006;18(1):41-50.

68. Vartanian JG, Carvalho AL, Carvalho SM, Mizobe L, Magrin J, Kowalski LP. Pectoralis major and other myofascial/myocutaneous flaps in head and neck cancer reconstruction: experience with 437 cases at a single institution. Head Neck. 2004;26(12):1018-23.

69. Salvatori P, Motto E, Paradisi S, Zani A, Podrecca S, Molinari R. Oromandibular reconstruction using titanium plate and pectoralis major myocutaneous flap. Acta Otorhinolaryngol ItaL 2007;27(5):227-32.

70. Croce A, Moretti A, D'Agostino L, Neri G. Continuing validity of pectoralis major muscle flap 25 years after its first application. Acta Otorhinolaryngol ItaL 2003;23(4):297-304.

71. Liu R, Gullane P, Brown D, Irish J. Pectoralis major myocutaneous pedicled flap in head and neck reconstruction: retrospective review of indications and results in 244 consecutive cases at the Toronto General Hospital. J OtolaryngoL 2001;30(1):34-40.

72. Chedid RS, J.C.; Faria, T.P.; Galvão, M.S.L.; Moraes, L.; Leal, P.R.; Dias, F.L. Craniofacial reconstruction with microsurgical flaps: Critical analysis. Rev Bras Cir Cabeça e Pescoço. 2009;38(2): 103-7.

73. Yang GC, B.; Gao, Y. . Forearm free skin flap transplantation. Nat Med J China. 1981;61:139-44.

74. McGregor IA. Fasciocutaneous flaps in intraoral reconstruction. Clin Plast Surg. 1985;12(3):453-61.

75. Song YG, Chen GZ, Song YL. The free thigh flap: a new free flap concept based on the septocutaneous artery. Br J Plast Surg. 1984;37(2):149- 59.

76. Zhou G, Zhang QX, Chen GY. The earlier clinic experience of the reverse-flow anterolateral thigh island flap. Br J Plast Surg. 2005;58(2): 160-4.

77. Luo S, Raffoul W, Luo J, Luo L, Gao J, Chen L, et al. Anterolateral thigh flap: A review of 168 cases. Microsurgery. 1999;19(5):232-8.

78. Drever JM. Total breast reconstruction with either of two abdominal flaps. Plast Reconstr Surg. 1977;59(2): 185-90.

79. Drever JM. The epigastric island flap. Plast Reconstr Surg. 1977;59(3):343-6.

80. Hartrampf CR, Jr, Black PW, Beegle PH, Jr. Breast reconstruction following mastectomy. J Med Assoe Ga. 1987;76(5):328-34.

81. Itoh Y, Arai K. The deep inferior epigastric artery free skin flap: anatomic study and clinical application. Plast Reconstr Surg. 1993;91(5):853-63; discussion 64.

82. Akinci M, Ay S, Kamiloglu S, Ercetin O. Lateral arm free flaps in the defects of the upper extremity--a review of 72 cases. Hand Surg. 2005;10(2- 3): 177-85.

83. Hara I, Gellrich NC, Duker J, Schon R, Nilius M, Fakler O, et al. Evaluation of swallowing function after intraoral soft tissue reconstruction with microvascular free flaps. Int J Oral Maxillofac Surg. 2003;32(6):593-9.

84. Hidalgo DA, Pusic AL. Free-flap mandibular reconstruction: a 10-year follow-up study. Plast Reconstr Surg. 2002;110(2):438-49; discussion 50-1.

85. Reece GP, Bengtson BP, Schusterman MA. Reconstruction of the pharynx and cervical oesophagus using free jejunal transfer. Clin Plast Surg. 1994;21(1): 125-36.

86. Seidenberg B, Rosenak SS, Hurwitt ES, Som ML. Immediate reconstruction of the cervical oesophagus by a revascularised isolated jejunal segment. Ann Surg. 1959; 149(2): 162-71.

87. Fisher SR, Cameron R, Hoyt DJ, Cole TB, Seigler HF, Meyers WC. Free jejunal interposition graft for reconstruction of the oesophagus. Head Neck. 1990; 12(2): 126-30.

88. Disa JJ, Pusic AL, Hidalgo DH, Cordeiro PG. Simplifying microvascular head and neck reconstruction: a rational approach to donor site selection. Ann Plast Surg. 2001 ;47(4):385-9.

89. Aki FEB, J.M.; Pinto, F.R.; Durazzo, M.D.; Cunha, A. S.; Filho, G.B.S.; Ferraz, A.R. Use of the forearm microsurgical flap in head and neck reconstruction: experience of 11 cases. Rev Assoe Med Bras. 2000;46(2).

90. Ariyan S. The pectoralis major myocutaneous flap. A versatile flap for reconstruction in the head and neck. Plast Reconstr Surg. 1979;63(1):73-81.

91. Mouthuy B, Schoofs M, Calteux N, Remacle M, Hamoir M, Van den Eeckhout J, et al. Myocutaneous flaps of the pectoralis major. Anatomy, technique and clinical applications. Acta chirurgica Belgium. 1984;84(5):283-92.

92. Yinde LAB, Rapaport A, Fava S, Andrade Sobrinho J, Denardin OVP, Carvalho MB. Limitations of the viability of the pectoralis major myocutaneous flap in the head and neck: a study of 72 cases. Rev Col Bras Cir. 1999;26(2):73-7.

93. Tincani AJ, Martins AS, Barreto G, Steck JH, Brandalise NA. Pedicled myocutaneous flap with pectoralis major for head and neck reconstruction. Rev Col Bras Cir. 1993;20(3):118-23.

94. Pickrell KL, Baker HM, Collins JP. Reconstructive surgery of the chest wall. Surg Gynecol Obstet. 1947;84(4):465-76.

95. McCraw JB, Dibbell DG, Carraway JH. Clinicai definition of independent

myocutaneous vascular territories. Plast Reconstr Surg. 1977;60(3):341-52.

96. McCraw JB, Dibbell DG. Experimental definition of independent myocutaneous vascular territories. Plast Reconstr Surg. 1977;60(2):212-20.

97. Brown RG, Fleming WH, Jurkiewicz MJ. An island flap of the pectoralis major muscle. Br J Plast Surg. 1977;30(2):161-5.

98. Sisson GA, Bytell DE, Becker SP. Mediastinal dissection--1976: indications and newer techniques. Laryngoscope. 1977;87(5 Pt 1):751-9.

99. Manktelow RT, McKee NH, Vettese T. An anatomical study of the pectoralis major muscle as related to functioning free muscle transplantation. Plast Reconstr Surg. 1980;65(5):610-5.

100. Pinto FR, Malena CR, Vanni CM, Capelli Fde A, Matos LL, Kanda JL. Pectoralis major myocutaneous flaps for head and neck reconstruction: factors influencing occurrences of complications and the final outcome. Sao Paulo Med J. 2010;128(6):336-41.

101. Arnold PG, Pairolero PC. Use of pectoralis major muscle flaps to repair defects of anterior chestwall. Plast Reconstr Surg. 1979;63(2):205-13.

102. Woods JE, Arnold PG, Masson JK, Irons GB, Payne WS. Management of radiation necrosis and advanced cancer of the chest wall in patients with breast malignancy. Plast Reconstr Surg. 1979;63(2):235-41.

103. Chaffai MA, Mansat M. Anatomic basis for the construction of a musculotendinous flap derived from the pectoralis major muscle. Surg Radiol Anat. 1988;10(4):273-82.

104. Bloch RJA, J.M.; Chem, R.C.; Azevedo, J.F. Atlas anatomo clínico dos retalhos musculares e miocutâneos. São Paulo1984.

105. Viterbo FP, J.C. Pectoralis major myocutaneous flap, anatomical study. Rev Bras Cir. 1985;75(4):229-36.

106. Testut LL, A. Tratado de anatomia humana. Barcelona1983.

107. Depaulis J, Colomb O. A case of congenital absence of the major pectoralis muscle. Ann Chir Plast. 1977;22(3):241-4.

108. Fokin AA, Robicsek F. Poland's syndrome revisited. Ann Thorac Surg. 2002;74(6):2218-25.

109. Ariyan S, Sasaki CT, Spencer D. Radical en bloc resection of the temporal bone. Am J Surg. 1981;142(4):443-7.

110. Ariyan S. Further experiences with the pectoralis major myocutaneous flap for the immediate repair of defects from excisions of head and neck cancers. Plast Reconstr Surg. 1979;64(5):605-12.

111. Urken MLB, H.F.; . Pectoralis major. In: Urken MLC, M.L.; Sillivan, M.J.; Biller, H.F., editor. Atlas of regional and free flaps for head and neck reconstruction. 1st ed. ed. New York: Raven Press; 1995. p. 3-28.

112. Yang D, Marshall G, Morris SF. Variability in the vascularity of the pectoralis major muscle. J Otolaryngol. 2003;32(1):12-5.

113. Cunha-Gomes D, Choudhari C, Kavarana NM. Vascular compromise of the pectoralis major musculocutaneous flap in head and neck reconstruction. Ann Plast Surg. 2003;51(5):450-4.

114. Pandey SK, Tripathi FM, Shukla VK, Tripathi CB, Sonoo J. Anatomical basis for the clinical application of the arterial supply of musculus pectoralis major. Acta Anat (Basel). 1991;141(4):302-6.

115. Friedrich W, Lierse W, Herberhold C. Myocutaneous vascular territory of the thoracoacromial artery. A topographical and morphometric study of the arterial vascularisation of the pectoralis major myocutaneous flap. Acta Anat (Basel). 1988;131(4):284-91.

116. Moloy PJ, Gonzales FE. Vascular anatomy of the pectoralis major myocutaneous flap. Arch Otolaryngol Head Neck Surg. 1986; 112(1):66-9.

117. Wei WI, Lam KH, Wong J. The true pectoralis major myocutaneous island flap: an anatomical study. Br J Plast Surg. 1984;37(4):568-73.

118. Reid CD, Taylor GL The vascular territory of the acromiothoracic axis. British journal of plastic surgery. 1984;37(2): 194-212.

119. Mathes SJ, Nahai F. Classification of the vascular anatomy of muscles: experimental

and clinicai correlation. Plast Reconstr Surg. 1981 ;67(2): 177-87.

120. Hoffman GW, Elliott LF. The anatomy of the pectoral nerves and its significance to the general and plastic surgeon. Annals of surgery. 1987;205(5):504-7.

121. Morain WD, Colen LB, Hutchings JC. The segmental pectoralis major muscle flap: a function-preserving procedure. Plast Reconstr Surg. 1985;75(6):825-30.

122. de Azevedo JF. Modified pectoralis major myocutaneous flap with partial preservation of the muscle: a study of 55 cases. Head Neck Surg. 1986;8(5):327-31.

123. Chen XH, Han DM, Huang ZG, Fang JG, Ni X, Zhou WG, et al. Application of modified pectoralis major myocutaneous island flap in head and neck surgeries. Zhonghua Er Bi Yan Hou Tou Jing Wai Ke Za Zhi. 2009;44(1):31-5.

124. Deo SV, Purkayastha J, Das DK, Kar M, Srinivas G, Asthana S, et al. Reconstruction of complex oral defects using bi-paddle pectoralis major flap - technical modifications and outcome in 54 cancer patients. Indian J Otolaryngol Head Neck Surg. 2003;55(1):5-9.

125. Simunovic F, Koulaxouzidis G, Stark GB, Torio-Padron N. Infraareolar pectoralis major myocutaneous island flap as treatment of first choice for deep sternal wound infection. J Plast Reconstr Aesthet Surg. 2013;66(2): 187-92.

126. Trignano E, Fallico N, Nitto A, Chen HC. The treatment of composite defect of bone and soft tissues with a combined latissimus dorsi and serratus anterior and RGB free flap. Microsurgery. 2013.

127. Kerawala CJ. Complications of head and neck cancer surgery - prevention and management. Oral OncoL 2010;46(6):433-5.

128. Carvalho AL, Miguel REV, Santos CR, Magrin J, Gonçalves Filho J, Kowalski LP. Total pharyngeal reconstruction: analysis of 69 cases. Rev Col Bras Cir. 1999;26(2):85-9.

129. Azevedo JF, Castro Júnior FM, Amora Filho MA, Cavalcante PI, Arraes RB. Pectoralis major myocutaneous flap in head and neck cancer repair surgery. Ceará Med. 1981;3(2):39-42.

130. Azevedo JF, Moura Filho MB, Farias JW, Trindade JW, Quixada PR, Frota MA. Immediate one-time reconstruction of the cervical oesophagus and hypopharynx with a modified pectoralis major isolated myocutaneous flap. Ceará Med. 1982;4(2):70-4.

131. Adekeye EO, Lavery KM, Nasser NA. The versatility of pectoralis major and latissimus dorsi myocutaneous flaps in the reconstruction of cancrum oris defects of children and adolescents. J Maxillofac Surg. 1986;14(2):99-102.

132. Belli E, Cicconetti A. The indications for reconstruction of the oral cavity using a pedicled flap of the musculus pectoralis major. Minerva stomatologica. 1994;43(4): 155-65.

133. Goldstein RD, Komisar A, Silver C, Strauch B. Management of necrotic neck wounds with a "sandwich" pectoralis myocutaneous flap. Head & neck surgery. 1988; 10(4):246-51.

134. Wilson JS. Recent advances in reconstruction in the head and neck region. Annals of the Academy of Medicine, Singapore. 1983; 12(2 Suppl):396- 401.

135. Sisson GA, Goldman ME. Pectoral myocutaneous island flap for reconstruction of stomal recurrence. Arch Otolaryngol. 1981;107(7):446-9.

136. Nakajima K, Ide Y, Abe S, Okada M, Kikuchi A, Ide Y. Anatomical study of the pectoral branch of thoracoacromial artery. The Bulletin of Tokyo Dental College. 1997;38(3):207-15.

137. Park HD, Min YS, Kwak HH, Youn KH, Lee EW, Kim HJ. Anatomical study concerning the origin and course of the pectoral branch of the thoracoacromial trunk for the pectoralis major flap. Surg Radiol Anat. 2004;26(6):428-32.

138. Cordeiro PG, Disa JJ. Challenges in midface reconstruction. Semin Surg Oncol. 2000; 19(3):218-25.

139. Futran ND, Mendez E. Developments in reconstruction of midface and maxilla. Lancet Oncol. 2006;7(3):249-58.

140. Rikimaru H, Kiyokawa K, Inoue Y, Tai Y. Three-dimensional anatomical vascular distribution in the pectoralis major myocutaneous flap. Plast Reconstr Surg. 2005; 115(5): 1342-52; discussion 53-4.

141. Daniel MM, Lorenzi MC, da Costa Leite C, Lorenzi-Filho G. Pharyngeal dimensions in healthy men and women. Clinics (Sao Paulo, Brazil). 2007;62(1):5-10.

142. Jemal A, Siegel R, Ward E, Hao Y, Xu J, Murray T, et al. Cancer statistics, 2008. CA: a cancer journal for clinicians. 2008;58(2):71-96.

143. Lore JM, Jr, Medina JE. An atlas of head and neck surgery. 4 ed. Philadelphia: Elsevier Saunders; 2005. 405-24 p.

144. NBR A. Tape measure - Natural or synthetic fibre - Specification. 10124:1987 Corrected Version: 1990 1987.

145. NBR A. Measuring and control instrument - Steel tape measure - Requirements. 10123:2012 2012.

146. de Matos LLV, C. M.; de Matos, M. G.; Kanda, J. L.; Brandão, L. G.; Pinto, F. R. The pectoral branch of the thoracoacromial artery as the main pedicle of the pectoralis major myocutaneous flap: an anatomical study in a cadaver. Rev Bras Cir Cabeça Pescoço. 2010;39(1):71 -6.

147. NBR A. Basic human body measurements for technical design. ISO 7250-1:2010 2010.

148. Vanni CM, Pinto FR, de Matos LL, de Matos MG, Kanda JL. The subclavicular versus the supraclavicular route for pectoralis major myocutaneous flap: a cadaveric anatomic study. Eur Arch OtorhinolaryngoL 2010;267(7):1141-6.

149. Chedid R, Sbalchiero JC, Farias TP, Galvão MSL, Moraes L, Leal PR, et al. Craniofacial reconstruction with microsurgical flaps: a critical analysis. Rev Bras Cir Cabeça Pescoço. 2009;38(2): 103-7.

150. Miyamoto S, Sakuraba M, Nagamatsu S, Kamizono K, Fujiki M, Hayashi R. Combined use of free jejunum and pectoralis major muscle flap with skin graft for reconstruction after salvage total pharyngolaryngectomy. Microsurgery. 2013;33(2): 119-24.

151. You YS, Chung CH, Chang YJ, Kim KH, Jung SW, Rho YS. Analysis of 120 pectoralis major flaps for head and neck reconstruction. Arch Plast Surg. 2012;39(5):522-7.

152. Dedivitis RA, Guimaraes AV. Pectoralis major musculocutaneous flap in head and neck cancer reconstruction. World J Surg. 2002;26(1):67-71.

153. Durazzo MD, Brandão LG. Complications of myocutaneous flaps: a review article. Rev Bras Cir Cabeça Pescoço. 2005;34(1):27-30.

154. Ribeiro Salles Vanni CM, de Matos LL, Faro Júnior MP, Ledo Kanda J, Cernea CR, Garcia Brandao L, et al. Enhanced morbidity of pectoralis major myocutaneous flap used

for salvage after previously failed oncological treatment and unsuccessful reconstructive head and neck surgery. ScientificWorldJournaL 2012;2012:384179.

155. Kroll SS, Evans GR, Goldberg D, Wang BG, Reece GP, Miller MJ, et al. A comparison of resource costs for head and neck reconstruction with free and pectoralis major flaps. Plast Reconstr Surg. 1997;99(5): 1282-6.

156. Castelli ML, Pecorari G, Sueco G, Bena A, Andreis M, Sartoris A. Pectoralis major myocutaneous flap: analysis of complications in difficult patients. Eur Arch Otorhinolaryngol. 2001;258(10):542-5.

157. de Bree R, Reith R, Quak JJ, Uyl-de Groot CA, van Agthoven M, Leemans CR. Free radial forearm flap versus pectoralis major myocutaneous flap reconstruction of oral and oropharyngeal defects: a cost analysis. Clin Otolaryngol. 2007;32(4):275-82.

158. Porcuna DV, Vintró LV, Vilas ML, Olmo AP, Ayala JM, Agustía MQ. Pectoralis major flaps. Evolution of their use in the age of microvascularised flaps. Acta otorrinolaringologica espanola. 2008;59(6):263-8.

159. Dubsky PC, Stift A, Rath T, Kornfehl J. Salvage surgery for recurrent carcinoma of the hypopharynx and reconstruction using jejunal free tissue

transfer and pectoralis major muscle pedicled flap. Arch Otolaryngol Head Neck Surg. 2007;133(6):551-5.

160. Qureshi SS, Ahmed QG, Yadav PS. Successful reconstruction of large oropharyngeal defect with pectoralis major myocutaneous flap in a four-year-old boy with recurrent fibromatosis. World J Surg Oncol. 2007;5:11.

161. Resto VA, McKenna MJ, Deschler DG. Pectoralis major flap in composite lateral skull base defect reconstruction. Arch Otolaryngol Head Neck Surg. 2007;133(5):490-4.

162. Zbar RI, Funk GF, McCulloch TM, Graham SM, Hoffman HT. Pectoralis major myofascial flap: a valuable tool in contemporary head and neck reconstruction. Head Neck. 1997;19(5):412-8.

163. Antunes AA, Antunes AP. Reconstruction of the exenterated orbital cavity: free skin graft or temporofrontal flap? Rev Cir Traumatol Buco-maxilo-fac. 2006;6(1):9-14.

164. Bianchi B, Ferri A, Ferrari S, Copelli C, Poli T, Sesenna E. Free and locoregional flap

associations in the reconstruction of extensive head and neck defects. International journal of oral and maxillofacial surgery. 2008;37(8):723-9.

165. Kovacevic P, Ugrenovic S, Kovacevic T. Vascularisation of pectoralis major myocutaneous flap: anatomical study in human fetuses and cadavers. Bosnian journal of basic medical sciences / Udruzenje basicnih mediciniskih znanosti = Association of Basic Medical Sciences. 2008;8(2): 183-7.

166. Candiani P, Campigliq GL, Quattrone P, Lovaria A. Computerised angiographic study of the vascular supply of the pectoralis major muscle. Acta Chir Plast. 1991 ;33(4): 185-93.

167. Kerawala CJ, Sun J, Zhang ZY, Guoyu Z. The pectoralis major myocutaneous flap: Is the subclavicular route safe? Head Neck. 2001;23(10):879-84.

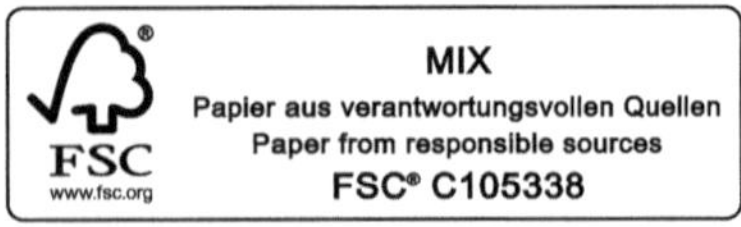

Printed by Books on Demand GmbH, Norderstedt / Germany